The Ten Habits of Naturally Slim People

And How to Make Them Part of Your Life

JILL H. PODJASEK, M.S., R.N.,
with JENNIFER CARNEY

CB
CONTEMPORARY BOOKS

Library of Congress Cataloging-in-Publication Data

Podjasek, Jill H.
    The ten habits of naturally slim people : and how to make them part
of your life / Jill H. Podjasek with Jennifer Carney.
        p.   cm.
    Includes bibliographical references and index.
    ISBN 0-8092-3177-8 (cloth)
    ISBN 0-8092-2953-6 (paper)
    1. Body image.   2. Leanness—Psychological aspects.
3. Mind and body.   4. Weight loss.   I. Carney, Jennifer.   II. Title.
BF697.5.B63P63   1997
613.2'5—dc21   97-6713
                                          CIP

Cover illustration by Jill Banashek
Interior design by Scott Rattray

Published by Contemporary Books
A division of NTC/Contemporary Publishing Group, Inc.
4255 West Touhy Avenue, Lincolnwood (Chicago), Illinois 60646-1975 U.S.A.
Printed in the United States of America
International Standard Book Number: 0-8092-3177-8 (cloth)
                                      0-8092-2953-6 (paper)
99 00 01 02 03 04 LB 19 18 17 16 15 14 13 12 11 10 9 8 7 6 5 4

To my teacher Bhagavan Sri Sathya Sai Baba
with love and devotion

May this book serve its readers
by teaching them to clear their minds,
open their hearts,
and be at peace with their bodies.

Sai Ram

Contents

Acknowledgments

WE WOULD LIKE to acknowledge the following people for the support and expertise they gave to us during this project: Betsy Schatz, R.N., wellness educator; Rob Williams, M.A., founder of the Psych-K Centre; Lisa Whaley, C.N., nutritionist; Brian Russell, fitness consultant/inventor; and Vic Martineau, graphic artist. Also a special thanks to Linda Gray, Senior Editor, for her continued faith in this project from the very first query letter.

Preface

THERE ARE CERTAIN landmarks by which we define periods of our lives. One 25-year period of my life began the day I went on my first diet and ended on the day I went on my last! At some time around the age of 18, I decided that I was fat. By the time I was 43, I had lost and gained thousands of pounds and was 75 pounds heavier than when I started. I wanted the weight off, and I was desperate. I wrote out a check for $300 and signed a contract with a diet program that gave me little packets of gruel to eat instead of meals. After three days, I threw all the little packets away and vowed I would never diet again. I had been dieting, and getting fatter, for almost 25 years. Either something was wrong with me or something was very wrong with the diet industry. Probably one of the healthiest decisions I ever made was deciding that the diet industry was screwed up, not I.

I'll never forget the first "antidiet" book I ever read, *How to Become Naturally Thin by Eating More* by Jean Antonello, R.N. It was clear and simple, and it gave me a sense that I was not alone in the world. However, on a daily basis I *was* alone. There were no antidiet programs, and even if there had been, I'm not sure I would have joined them anyway. I wasn't on a vendetta *against* dieting; I was just *for* something else. I longed to discuss with someone what I was trying to do, but I wasn't even sure myself. Around this time I met Jennifer Carney, a renegade from the diet industry, who was teaching exactly what I was trying to do myself.

Before Jennifer left her job as an instructor for a major weight loss program, she had kept 70 pounds off for five years by keeping a food diary every single day, starving during the week, and bingeing on weekends. She finally left the industry for the same reasons I did. Something was wrong—losing weight should not be so debilitating! Jennifer started a program called "Say NO to DIETS, Say YES to LIFE!," threw her food diaries away, and began to study the habits of naturally slim people. We joined together on a mission of the heart; she a psychiatric nurse turned motivational speaker and I a critical care nurse turned writer. We have collaborated on several projects.

Just by beginning to believe that there wasn't something "wrong" or "bad" about us because we struggled with our weight, that we were normal and that we were born with all the natural abilities of everyone else, we began to eat differently and lose weight. It became clear to us in our studies that the answer to becoming slim for life was to rediscover all of the positive natural attributes that we already have working in our favor. We must unlock our own potential and put it into action, not follow blindly the dictates of a book or program. For this book we conducted observations of and interviews with naturally slim people from all walks of life, and we sent out questionnaires to naturally slim people all over the country. We define a naturally slim person as a person who has never dieted and who maintains a steady healthy weight without obsessions about food or exercise. The information and insight gained from these people is invaluable, and it is the basis of this book's philosophies on how all of us can become naturally slim.

Nobody gains or loses weight in the exact same way or for the exact same reasons, however. Each journey to health and slimness is individual. The person most capable of individualizing your program is you! You know yourself better than anyone else possibly can. If you don't, then your very first step toward health will be to develop an awareness and understanding of yourself and your thoughts, feelings, beliefs, and actions.

Many of the ideas presented in this book are not completely new. The *truth* is ancient and universal. It will continue to resurface in different ways and be clothed in different words throughout time. We thank the many pioneers who have gone before us in presenting ideas concerning natural weight loss. It is our hope that this time around, as the century turns and paradigms shift, millions of people who have been at war with their bodies will be ready to embrace the truth—that we already have a blueprint for slimness within us. All we need to do is take the time to dust it off, understand it, and build!

Jill Herrmann Podjasek

I am fascinated by the power of words and their meanings. I had been studying them and working on my definition of *self* long before my adventures through obesity and slimness. What I have discovered is that being slim has more to do with knowing who you are than knowing what to eat. In fact, when you know who you are you will naturally know what to eat. We are not born to blow up and self-destruct; we are born to live. What most of us don't even realize is that we have certain birthrights. I remind myself daily that I was born with self-esteem, that I was born with a self-regulating body, that I was born with hunger and satiety signals, and that I was born with the right to determine how I live my life.

It is by acknowledging and understanding these birthrights that you will be able to activate them in your life. May you enjoy and savor the experience of this book and then bless yourself with all of the time and love you need to become the real you, in spirit, mind, and body.

Bon Appétit!
Jennifer Carney

Introduction

WE INVITE YOU now to step out of the process of dieting and into the process of health. To discover your natural ability to be healthy and slim without food plans, exercise regimes, deprivation, or willpower. To know that you are normal and that the state of your physical body is merely a manifestation of years of imbalance—of the body, the mind, and the spirit. If you are willing to explore them, your food, weight, and body issues can serve as a gateway to self-discovery that will improve your entire life, not just the size of your body.

When choosing to change and learn new ways of doing things, it is helpful to choose a master or role model to observe. A role model serves as a touchstone for truth in practice as you are learning. He or she should be an outstanding example of the thoughts, words, and actions that you wish to make part of your life. In the past you may have followed the example or teachings of those who struggle with their bodies and work very hard to stay slim. Now you can choose a different model, the model of the naturally slim person. We all came into this world naturally slim, which makes following this model like coming home.

Books and programs that are based solely on actions such as counting fat grams and relentlessly exercising rarely lead to permanent weight loss. Changing the attitudes, thoughts, and beliefs behind these physical actions will. This is what makes this book such a valuable tool for improving your life and your weight.

If you have come to this book looking for a quick fix or a magic food plan, you have come to the wrong place. Losing weight permanently is a process of growth and change. There are several steps to this process. If you skip steps you may get quick weight loss but you won't get permanent weight loss. You will short-change your own future by thinking that losing a certain amount of weight must be done by a certain date. Whether this is your first or your 15th book about losing weight, *please* give yourself the gift of time. The key to success is to take all the time you need to learn and practice and focus on the process, not the pounds.

What Is the Process of Growth and Change?

The process of growth and change is a series of steps we must go through in order to think and act in a new way. The basic steps are:

Awareness: waking up, feeling, seeing, touching, hearing internally and externally. Being alert, paying attention not just to physical experiences but also to mental, emotional, and spiritual experiences.

Introspection: thinking about your "self," about your thoughts, your feelings, your actions and reactions, your wants, and your needs.

Letting Go of the Past: acknowledging the past that contributed to where you are today and then letting it go in order to move forward. This involves grieving for what you are leaving behind.

Acceptance of Self and Others: a sense of peace about who you are and where you are and an absence of anger and blame for your current state of body and mind.

Embracing Change: an attitude that learning about yourself is enjoyable and that mistakes are not bad, but rather the foundation for learning. A true commitment to moving forward and being different from how you were.

Willingness to be in the process of growing instead of being done. You're ready to take action and to do the work necessary to move forward.

Growth: a progressive development of the self toward a higher, more fulfilling, level of living.

Increased Awareness: as you grow, your awareness and consciousness increase, allowing you to perceive other thoughts, feelings, and actions, often uncomfortable, and leading you to further **introspection.**

As you can see, the process cycles back to the beginning. As long as you stay in the process, you will continue to grow and improve your life and your weight. This process is not always fast, and it is not always smooth, but if you stay in it, taking one *small* step at a time, the rewards can be tremendous.

Where Do I Start and What Do I Do?

Start by taking your first small step in the area of *awareness*. You choose what step and how big. You can decide to be more awake to everything in your life, or you may choose one specific area of your life. You might choose to do one of the awareness exercises found in this book. From your increased awareness choose one small, specific thing you have noticed that gives you discomfort that you would like to feel different about. For example, maybe you've become aware that putting on clothes that are too tight for you upsets you.

Instead of jumping into the whole "I need to lose weight" scenario, every time you get dressed, take a small step into *introspection*. Contemplate what you really think and feel about your tight clothes. Notice all the emotions a single piece of inanimate cloth can drag up. Notice the stream of negative thoughts you have about how fat you are, how ugly you are, how you don't deserve to get any new clothes until you lose weight, and the painful memories of your last 10 unsuccessful diets. Look closely at these thoughts. Is there one particular thought you could change that would keep you from getting depressed every time you get dressed? How about "I don't deserve to get any new clothes until I lose weight." This is not true. You deserve to have clothes that allow you to be comfortable as you work and play. Clothes are not meant to be a punishment.

The next step is to *let go of the old* thought and *embrace the new*. Start telling yourself every day, "I deserve to have comfortable clothes to wear." At first you may not be able to say this without cringing, but gradually you will begin to own the statement and believe it. This is the beginning of *accepting yourself* at the size you are. Soon you will be highly motivated to get yourself comfortable clothes no matter what size they are. Getting dressed in the morning can begin to become pleasurable instead of painful.

This is just one example of being in the process of growth and change. You can and will create hundreds of your own examples, personalized to you and your particular body, mind, and spirit. The Process of Growth and Change is discussed in more detail in Chapter 20. You may find it helpful to read Chapter 20 before you read the rest of the book.

Using "Opportunities for Growth"

At the end of most chapters there is a section called "Opportunities for Growth." These opportunities will assist you in putting into action the material presented in each chapter. The "Awareness" section contains activities designed to wake up your senses and challenge perceptions you may have about yourself and your environment. The "Introspection" section offers activities that encourage you to look inside yourself, and to ask yourself questions about how you think and feel. Next are "Old Beliefs to Let Go." These are beliefs that keep you from your slim nature. After the old beliefs we list a set of "New Beliefs to Embrace." These are beliefs that support the process of becoming naturally slim.

The old and new beliefs included in the section are samples of the most common beliefs we run across in our practice. The list is not all-inclusive; you can personalize it by adding your own beliefs. In the second half of the book you will learn how to assimilate new beliefs into your subconscious using psychological kinesiology, a highly reliable and measurable technique for incorporating positive new beliefs into our lives. Until then you can begin to embrace new beliefs by repeating them face to face with yourself in a mirror or by writing and reading them several times a day. In general, if a chapter does not have an "Opportunities for Growth" section it is because that chapter provides information that will assist you overall in your growth.

The "Vividly Imagine" section provides a jumping-off point for you to create your own vivid imagery. When creating your images, write them down, be as vivid with details as possible, use words that are meaningful to you (use the dictionary to embel-lish), and read and visualize the images you created in detail at least once a day. Tape-recording the visualization is even better, because you can sit with your eyes closed and listen, focusing on the visualization itself instead of on reading the words. If you decide to make a tape, be sure to speak slowly and to allow time for your mind to fully form pictures of the images you wish to create.

"Patterns for Action" is the last section. Don't rush into this section. It is very important to set up your foundation for change mentally, with beliefs and images, before you attempt to take even the smallest physical action. The actions we suggest are purposely the very smallest of changes to get you rolling. You may not be ready for these for a while. After you have these beginning changes entrenched as habits, you can build the next level of action yourself from the information in the book.

"Additional Reading" provides the names of books and chapters with valuable information that will allow you to explore topics of your choice in depth. These books have been chosen specifically because they are harmonious with our philosophies. However, that does not mean the entire book agrees with us. When in doubt, we suggest you return to this book for validation. Occasionally we run across a book with helpful information in the front and a standard, unrealistic diet plan in the back. Please ignore any diets or food plans in the additional readings.

Reading for Results

This book is very different from books you may have read on the subject of losing weight. Many books take a look at only one small part of the multifaceted nature of weight loss. Examples of this are books that address only fat grams or only exercise or only emotional eating. We have chosen instead to provide you with a comprehensive guide concerning the many issues that confront people on a daily basis as they try to lose weight. You will be given new information about becoming slim *and* the tools you need to incorporate that information into your life.

This is a formidable goal to take on in one book. However, we believe that the majority of our readers are ready for something different and are willing to become students of the Naturally Slim weight loss process. Being a student means that you become responsible for your own learning. You may take notes as you read; you can even write down questions and forward them to us (see back page for the address). You will probably read certain chapters more than once.

To get the most out of all of the information in this book we encourage you to see it as an ongoing resource to consult as you change and grow. There are many ways to do this. You can read the book cover to cover, skipping over the "Opportunities for Growth" sections, then go back and work through them later. Or you can read slowly, doing each exercise as you go along. If you don't care for exercises you may choose to read the book and glean from it what you can without doing any of them.

There are as many different ways to read and use this book as there are readers who read it. The best advice we can give you is to take your time, take small bites, and enjoy what you're doing. If you are feeling overwhelmed or overworked you are trying to do too much too fast. If you feel that nothing is happening, maybe you're doing too little. Taking the smallest of steps in a forward direction is the surest way to keep in the process. Look at your success in each step that you take rather than judging your progress by your weight. A lot will happen in your heart and your head before anything shows up on the scale.

Read *The Ten Habits of Naturally Slim People*, then take the opportunity to grow and make them part of your life!

ONE

Diet Mentality: The Mind-Body Connection That Keeps You Fat

The state of your mind is more important to reaching a state of health than diet or exercise. It is your subconscious and conscious mind working in unison that will either support you or sabotage you on your journey.

OVER THE LAST century the popular definition of the word *diet* has changed dramatically. In the past the word meant simply "...what a living being eats for sustenance," as in "A bird's *diet* consists mainly of seeds and berries." In today's world the word *diet* has the power to evoke shivers, cringes, and severe mental anguish. Today *diet* most often refers to any one of 1,000 plans or programs that require restriction and monitoring of food intake for the purpose of losing weight—as in "I can't eat that; I'm on a *diet*." Being on a diet or dieting fosters an altered state of mind that we refer to as "diet mentality." The scary part of the diet mentality is that it does not necessarily disappear when a person stops dieting. In fact this altered state of mind usually becomes an integral part of the person's everyday thinking. Diet mentality is a state of mind that affects not only the way you perceive your body and the food you nourish it with but also the way you perceive your whole self: body, mind, and spirit.

Americans spend over $32 billion a year on diets and diet-related products. Money well spent if it led to creating permanent, healthy changes in our lives. But it hasn't. America remains the fattest nation on earth, with an eight-pound gain in the weight of the average American over the last 10 years. The key word here is *permanent*. The multibillion-dollar diet industry is built on repeat customers. If diet programs resulted in permanent weight loss for their clients, the programs would put themselves out of business. In any given year, approximately 75 percent of those joining commercial weight loss programs are repeat customers! Why do we continue to do the same thing over and over again, expecting different results? It is now very widely published that anywhere from 95 to 98 percent of people who lose weight on a diet gain all that weight back within five years. It is very likely that 98 percent of the people picking up this book have lived those statistics more than once! Almost all of us have dieted, and almost all of us have lost; lost time, lost money, lost health, lost energy, lost our ability to metabolize normally, lost muscle mass, lost self-esteem, and lost hope that we may ever feel or look good again.

Does any diet work? Yes, almost all of them do—temporarily. Diets are very successful at producing temporary weight loss and all the temporary good feelings that go along with it. However, physiologically and psychologically almost every diet is doomed to fail. Physiologically, severe restrictions in food intake trigger in our bodies what is called a *famine mode*. To guarantee our survival, when the body senses a famine it (1) slows down its metabolism; (2) conserves energy and readily stores fat; and (3) burns muscle as well as fat when it runs out of available calories. This combination causes us to lose calorie-burning power with every bit of muscle that is lost and to burn fewer calories and store fat more easily when we go off the diet. Each subsequent diet compounds these effects. This is why a person can start dieting at 150 pounds and then 10 diets and 10 years later weigh 200 pounds. This is in spite of the fact that the diets were temporarily "successful" and that the dieter is eating *less* food at 200 pounds than she or he did at 150 pounds!

The effects are also devastating psychologically. When the fleeting success of the diet wanes and the pounds start creeping back on no matter how "good" you are, panic sets in. Panic is followed by guilt. Guilt is followed by body hate and sometimes starving and bingeing. Anger and self-recrimination may turn into an "I can do this" burst of strength. But alas, this burst of strength is used to go on yet another new and improved diet, and the cycle starts all over again. This diet → weight loss → weight-gain → diet cycle, sometimes called *yo-yo dieting*, is not at all benign. In the representation in Figure 1 you can see that this is not just a cycle; it is an insidious downward spiral. A cycle is rather like a merry-go-round. You can choose to ride it once or you can choose to ride it 50 times, but either way, when you choose to get off you will be exactly where you started. In the case of dieting, going around even once can leave your self-esteem, your muscle mass, and your metabolism at a lower point than where you started. Each time you go around again you start at a lower point and end up even lower.

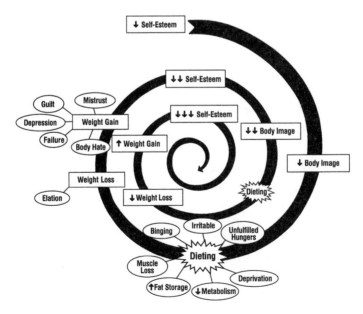

Figure 1. The Self-Defeating Spiral of Yo-Yo Dieting

A Conversation with Diet Mentality

I am Diet Mentality, an insidious mind-set belonging to those of you who are constantly at war with your body. I start out as a gentle ripple in your thoughts, a glance in the mirror, a look of disapproval, and the first diet is cast. With each and every diet, the thoughts rapidly grow in force and speed, a vortex circling downward. A black hole that sucks the spirit out of those of you who diet and hate and diet and hate. I feed on your self-doubt; I feed on your fears and insecurities. Possessed by the idea that you need to change your body to be OK, you reach out to one more diet and are sucked into my thoughts ever more deeply.

I urge you to constantly look outside yourself for answers. I convince you that you are weak and cannot find the answers in yourself. Not knowing what else to do, you reach out to dieting, starving, exercising over and over again. Thoughts of your imperfect body cloud every moment of the day, crowding out any thoughts of happiness and joy. You see a thin reflection in my pond and, grasping for the image, tumble head over heels into my putrid waters. There is a stench about me, a stench of death, of spirits lost: anorexics, bulimics, the morbidly obese, the starved, the stapled, the liposuctioned . . . Globs of hated fat are strewn throughout my waters.

To you who think my thoughts, a thin body is a god and a diet an offering to that god: "Oh dear god of the eternally thin body, If I starve myself, if I exercise relentlessly, if I'm good and follow to the letter this 30-day plan, wilt thou look favorably upon me and bless me with a thin body forever?" "Of course I will," he laughs, "but only if you are willing to give me your spirit. Only if you vow to live a life totally dedicated to physical perfection."

"I agree," says the dieter. "I agree to give up my spirit, my free will, my every waking thought, my happiness and peace of mind. I agree to follow all of the tenets of diet mentality in exchange for the eternally thin body."

The Tenets of Diet Mentality

My worth as a human being is determined solely by
the shape of my body.

•

I must at all times know what I weigh, and the quality
of each day is determined by the number on my
bathroom scale.

•

I am unable to decide on my own when, where, what, and
how much to eat. That must be determined for me by a diet.

•

Having an appetite is bad. I must suppress my appetite at all
costs, and when willpower is not enough I will use drugs,
fiber, methylcellulose—whatever works.

•

I should never feel hungry because if I do I might
eat uncontrollably.

•

There are GOOD foods and BAD foods. I should never
eat bad foods.

•

If I do eat a bad food, I should feel guilty and ashamed.

•

A reward means cheating on my diet.

•

If I go off my diet, I am a weak-willed cheater.

•

If I don't lose weight on my diet, there is something
wrong with me, not the diet.

If I gain weight, I am bad.

•

If I do not lose weight, I should punish myself.

•

I need a diet program director to tell me when I've been bad
and to pat me on the back when I am good.

•

I am loved only for the shape and size of my body.

•

I must live in constant fear that my body will blow up
like a big, fat balloon.

•

My life must revolve around the shape and size of my body,
food, diets, and exercise.

•

I must at all times hate my body and all of its imperfections.

HATE. That is what Diet Mentality feeds on:

Body hate

Insecurity

Fear

Mistrust

Ignorance

Low self-esteem

*I am Diet Mentality. I clutter your mind so that you
lose touch with who you truly are.*

*If you are in touch with your spirit, you cannot think
my thoughts.*

Dieting is a false prophet and thinness a false god. They offer nothing of lasting value.

You have everything you need to know within you. Everything, that is, except knowing that you know.

How do we get out of this spiral? How do we get out of this way of thinking? If we think differently, can we still become slim, or do we have to settle for fat and happy? Can we recover the health and self-love that we have lost? The answers are in this book. The most important step you can take now is to step out of the spiral. No matter how large you are or how low your spirit is, decide to step out of the process of dieting and into the process of health. Dieting has given you nothing. Be willing to do something different. That something is to become naturally slim.

The key to getting out of the diet mentality is to develop a whole new mentality to replace it—the mentality of a naturally slim person. Look to the people who are masters at being slim. The ones who have never dieted and who have been slim all their lives. Don't just be envious. Watch them. They think and act in ways that keep them healthy and slim, ways that you have long forgotten. They are masters of the art of slimness. They do not look to books and magazines to tell them what to eat. Their choices of food and exercise come naturally. Their moves are part of a mind-body-spirit connection that allows them to participate in their own health every moment of every day without a second thought.

How and when did you get sucked into the diet mentality? The time and place were different for each of us. For some of us it started when we were young children; for some of us it was in adolescence or at college. Others did not start dieting until they had children or reached middle age. However, one thing I know for sure. None of you were born thinking and eating the way you do now. Going back and understanding the way you thought and acted as a child can give you some very good lessons in what we call *natural, instinctive eating*—that is, choosing and eating foods instinctively, without guidelines or restrictions.

Opportunities for Growth

Awareness

- When did you go on your first diet? Why? What were you thinking about yourself when you went on it?

- When did you go on your last diet? Why? What were you thinking about yourself when you went on it?

- Plot a general graph of your weight since you started dieting. Do you weigh more now than when you first started dieting?

- Do you know people who have never dieted or who have tried dieting once but couldn't stick to it? Have they been at a healthy body weight most of their lives? Ask if you can talk to them about how they think and how they choose food and amounts.

Introspection

- What do you need to do to convince yourself that another diet won't work and you are ready for something different?

Old Beliefs to Let Go

- Every one of the "Tenets of Diet Mentality" is a belief to be let go. Read the tenets over. How many of them do you own? Can you think of any more beliefs you've acquired through chronic dieting? Write them down.

New Beliefs to Embrace

- I am ready, willing, and able to welcome change and growth into my life now.

- I willingly release my preoccupation with food, weight, and body size.

- I am now in the process of health.

Vividly Imagine

- Imagine how you might feel mentally, physically, and emotionally if you were not barraged with diet mentality thoughts all day long.

Patterns for Action

- Take mostly mental action right now. Begin to appreciate the value of awareness and introspection. Be willing to make them part of your everyday thinking.

- If you feel like doing something physical, take any or all of the tenets of diet mentality and rewrite them as positive, present-tense statements that support your desire to think in a different way. These positive statements will become New Beliefs to Embrace.

Additional Reading

Munter, Carol, and Jane Hirschman. *Overcoming Overeating.* New York: Fawcett Columbine, 1989.

Schwartz, Bob. *Diets Don't Work.* Las Vegas: Breakthru, 1986.

Stacy, Michelle. *Consumed—Why Americans Love, Hate and Fear Food.* New York: Simon and Schuster, 1994.

Triboli, Evelyn, M.S., R.D., and Elyse Resch, M.S., R.D. *Intuitive Eating.* New York: St. Martin's Press, 1995.

Two

Infants and Children: Slim by Nature

All of us were born to be healthy and naturally slim. The fact that you are not slim and healthy now merely means you have walked, perhaps for many years, away from your natural instincts.

PICTURE IN YOUR MIND a healthy, smiling infant. Imagine the smoothness of the baby's skin, all the little wrinkles and dimples. Touch his sensitive mouth. Look at the curiosity in his eyes. His tiny fingers reach out to grasp the world, ready to take in everything and anything without judgment. His first world of exploration is his very own body. He can spend hours looking at his own fingers or reaching for the toes on the end of his own foot, the joy of learning interrupted only by the need for food or water or sleep. The baby feels discomfort, maybe a pain in his stomach, and he cries out to be fed.

Thus his lessons about the outside world begin. If his cries are heard and he is comforted and fed, he begins to learn that the universe is a friendly place. If his cries are unheeded, fears and doubts begin to form. The totality of this baby's world is a pure drive to survive, thrive, and grow; to seek the feelings of joy, comfort, and love. Ahhh, you may be thinking, how sweet, how innocent, how unaffected by the world around him. No wonder he's happy.

Guess what? You are that baby! I am that baby! Each and every one of us was born with all the same wonderful instincts as that baby. We have just spent many years burying them under thousands of thoughts and beliefs. Hundreds of life experiences have dealt blows to our self-love, our trust, and our desire to grow. But these drives and instincts are not gone. They are forever a part of our nature as human beings. The challenge is to uncover them and allow them to be a guiding force in your journey to health and slimness. Using the infant and young child as a model, let's take a look at how their natural instincts guide them in their eating and exercise.

A Baby Eats Only When Hungry

When a baby feels irritable or her stomach is gnawing with emptiness, she *knows* she must eat. Hunger signals are inborn, attention-getting messages that guarantee we will seek food and stay alive. When a baby feels hungry, she does whatever she has to do to get food. This is a kind and loving thing to do for herself. Unfortunately, she must rely on people outside herself to meet those needs, and it is here that her expectations and beliefs about hunger, food, and satiety begin to be formed. In the beginning she feels hunger, she cries, and someone shows up with dinner. (Boy, I wish I could do that!) Basically, she eats when she is hungry.

A Baby Stops Eating When She Is Satisfied

When a baby has had enough to eat, she stops. She falls into a blissful sleep of satisfaction and delight. Have you ever tried to force a baby to take more milk than she wants? First, you would need a car jack to pry her mouth open. Then, if you do succeed in getting a few more drops in, she will spit them right back at you. She may be hungry again in two or three hours, at which time she will cry again, eat, become satisfied, and then stop eating. Eating every two or three hours may be inconvenient for the parents, but the baby will develop her own natural feeding schedule according to her nutritional needs if she is left alone. Some parents try to train their children out of eating so often. They may insist they wait four hours between feedings or eat only three meals a day. This sends many negative messages to the child: "When you're hungry, you won't always get food, so maybe you'd better eat more than you need in case you don't get any more." "The universe is an unfriendly place, and you may be in pain, but there are no guarantees that anyone will hear you." "You can't always trust your parents—they might feed you when you're hungry, or they might not." I encourage all of you, parents or not, to read some of the books about feeding and children listed at the end of this chapter.

If we go back to the time before our imaginary parents interfered with our imaginary baby's instincts, we see that a baby stops eating when satisfied. He does this regardless of what his parents think, and it does not matter to him whether he ate one hour ago or six hours ago. He operates on pure, natural, unadulterated instinct.

A baby does not:

> eat to keep from feeling hungry
>
> eat when bored
>
> eat when tired
>
> eat because Mom prepared the food
>
> eat because everyone else is eating
>
> eat because it's there
>
> eat because it's mealtime

Or eat for any of the thousands of other reasons we have invented—all of which reveal how unnatural our relationship with food, hunger, and satisfaction has become.

Preschoolers Show Us Their Instincts, Too

Let's age this imaginary baby a little bit. Imagine a toddler or pre-schooler, getting into everything, as curious as ever; running, jumping, climbing, learning to say no. Picture this young child with a plate of food in front of her. Maybe it has some peas on it, a couple of squares of cheese, some spiral noodles, and a few carrot sticks. First, her innate pleasure in discovery will drive her to play with the brightly colored food. She may make quite a mess before she begins to eat. If the child is truly hungry, she will eat the food her body needs the most, and she will then continue to eat different things until satisfied. She eats with joy and playful-ness—sucking the twisty noodles through her lips, bouncing the peas and then rolling them around on her tongue before she squishes them, turning each block of cheese into an indentured piece of art and making loud crunching noises as she bites the carrot sticks. She is experiencing food with a joie de vivre that many of us could learn from. Food is cool; food is fun; eating is a grand sensory experience! The toddler may throw the things she doesn't like to the floor or just push them away, but she will absolutely refuse to let a food she dislikes cross her lips. (Young children are often called picky eaters by their parents. I say hooray—be picky and stay picky!) When the child's physical hunger is satisfied, she will play with what's left on her plate until she is removed from the table.

Parents worry, often needlessly, about their child's nutrition during these years. Actually, it has been documented that young children do quite well nutritionally if left alone. That is, a small child who is given a wide variety of foods to choose from every day will consume a very balanced diet when measured over two weeks.

You are that child! All of us have within us the natural instincts to consume a healthy, nutritious, balanced diet. All of us are innately picky eaters. Granted, these instincts may be buried under pounds of well-meaning advice that we took to be truth, such as "Clean your plate or you don't get dessert," and "You took a second serving, and now you must eat it whether you are hungry or not," and "Don't eat now, or you will spoil your dinner," and above all, "Don't play with your food!"

A child:

eats when hungry

is very picky about what he eats

enjoys his food

stops eating when satisfied

Babies and young children are naturally slim because they are in touch with their natural drives and instincts.

There are many other things we can learn from these naturally slim little people: When you are tired, lie down and rest. When you are thirsty, drink water. Follow your natural drive toward pleasure and away from pain. Walking, running, jumping, dancing, and skipping rope are fun. When you are playing, play; when you are working, work; and when you are looking at a caterpillar, look at a caterpillar. One activity is no more valuable than the other. The value of an activity is lost only when we are not totally involved in it in body, mind, and spirit.

Remember, instincts cannot be lost. We are born with them, and they stay with us until we die. Our life experiences have trained us away from our natural instincts, but we can reawaken them by opening the doors of our hearts and minds, clearing a path for them, and practicing. How do you do this? Through this book you can reacquaint yourself with your own instincts by witnessing what naturally instinctive children and adults do. With your newly acquired knowledge you can practice the actions of these masters. At the same time you will learn how to clear self-defeating thoughts from your mind, allowing you easy access to your natural instincts. If you read, if you believe, if you practice, you too can join the ranks of the naturally slim. Because this is a process of permanent change based on your true nature, it will be yours for the rest of your life. The process is quite fun if you allow it to be. As you begin to take responsibility for yourself and your actions, you will be driven, like a detective, into your own mind to search for the release all the mental blocks you may have to becoming slim and healthy.

Opportunities for Growth

Awareness

- Keep your eyes open for opportunities to observe infants and children eating. Notice what they do and notice their attitudes toward different foods. How long does it take them to finish a meal? What are their parents' reactions to their eating? Can you pick out things that are being said to them that might encourage them to lose touch with their natural instincts about food? Hunger? Satisfaction?

Introspection

- Recall mealtimes at your house as you were growing up. What were they like? What were the rules? What were your parents' attitudes about food, cleaning your plate, dessert, and so forth?

- Do you see yourself still following those rules now as an adult? Are they rules that support your natural instincts? Or are they rules it would be better to abandon?

Old Beliefs to Let Go

The following are some childhood beliefs that you may want to let go of:

- It is good and healthy to clean your plate.

- Always eat what is put in front of you.

- It is bad to play with your food.

- Disregard your hunger and eat only when you're told.

New Beliefs to Embrace

The best new beliefs to embrace are those that you have discovered by rewriting your own old beliefs into positive, present-tense statements. Here are three that we have written:

- I have all of the natural instincts I was born with available to me right now.

- Eating according to my natural instincts is healthy and slimming.

- Learning to eat naturally again is a great adventure.

Vividly Imagine

- Pick a day, half a day, or even a few hours and view the world through the eyes of a child. Be sure to include a meal in there just for fun. Begin to become aware of the child-like parts of you that you have lost touch with: the part of you that likes to have fun; the part that only wants to eat exactly what you want; the part of you that is hungry *now* and doesn't want to wait until "lunchtime"; the part of you that likes to play with your food; the curious part of you that can spend an hour watching pigeons eat bread crumbs without judging them as dirty, disease-carrying, flying rats. Feel things physically and emotionally. Get out of your rut and wake up to the joy of just being.

Patterns for Action

- Take mostly mental action right now. Become involved in awareness and introspection.

- If you feel like doing something physical, begin a journal to record your new awareness and insight. Try writing down some of your most vivid recollections about your childhood mealtimes. If the recollections stimulate negative emotions, create new versions that are exactly how you would have liked it to be.

Additional Reading

Hirschman, Jane, and Lela Zaphiropoulos. *Solving Your Child's Eating Problems.* New York: Fawcett Columbine, 1985.

Satter, Ellyn. *How to Get Your Kid to Eat . . . But Not Too Much.* Palo Alto: Bull, 1987.

THREE

Naturally Versus Unnaturally Slim Adults

Ultimately what most people desire is health, happiness, and a long, productive life; not slimness at any cost. If you spend every waking moment striving for some esoteric standard of physical perfection, haven't you missed a good portion of your life?

YOU ARE NORMAL, and don't let anyone tell you any different! You were born with all the natural instincts of any other child born on this planet. Yes, you may have a genetic tendency toward a certain body type or a certain metabolism that precludes your being a six-foot-tall, waif-thin fashion model. However, you are definitely normal, and you were not born to be obese. We are not saying this to conjure up guilt in you because at this particular time you are overweight or obese. We are saying this because we want you to know that you have all the raw material necessary to develop a long, productive, happy, and healthy life. As you develop that life for yourself, slimness will be a naturally occurring part of it.

You may be thinking, if everyone has these wonderful natural instincts, why are some people fat and some people slim? And if we are all the same underneath, I want to be one of the slim ones! We agree with you; we want to be one of the slim ones too! That is how our research on naturally slim people started. We wanted to be slim, and we believed it didn't have to be difficult. In the tradition of the martial arts, we embarked on a journey to find a master whom we could study: someone who was slim and had been all his or her life, someone who was able to stay slim with very little effort, someone who could be our role model in thought and deed—a master in the art of natural slimness.

We began our search with friends and relatives and quickly moved on to acquaintances and strangers. We looked for people who had slim physical bodies, and we interviewed them about their lifestyles and about their eating habits. We also shared meals with them and watched how they ate. We asked them about how they shopped and cooked and exercised. We found that in the realm of being slim, outward appearances can be very deceiving. Most slim people fell into one of two categories, the naturally slim and the unnaturally slim. During our research, it became apparent to us that balance and health were qualities consistent with being naturally slim, whereas unnaturally slim people seemed out of balance and stressed.

Slim, but at What Price?

We chose the term *unnaturally slim* for this second group because we felt that they used unnatural amounts of willpower and control in the areas of food selections and exercise. They often used over-the-counter diuretics, appetite suppressants, or meal supplements to get to and remain in their slim state. Being and staying slim occupied most of their time and most of their thoughts. Although these people had the magazine and television version of an ideal body, they often saw their bodies as far from perfect. When asked what their secret to remaining slim was, they answered "hard work." The unnaturally slim laboriously monitor their eating, especially fat grams, and make sure that they "pay" for every indiscretion with exercise. Often they have elaborate exercise routines that last one to three hours per day.

The minds of the unnaturally slim were continuously occu-pied with the issues that surrounded maintaining their perfect bodies, yet they had little respect for their true needs: "No time for breakfast. I've got to go to the gym before work." Lunchtime arrives, and it's "I'm really hungry, but I should just have a salad or some yogurt." After work, "Gosh, those hors d'oeuvres look good, but they are so fattening, I think I'll pass." Then they chug down two or three glasses of wine to relieve the tension. Most of these people lived lives of quiet or not-so-quiet obsession and fear—fear of what would happen to them if they ever got fat. Their topics of conversation at coffee, lunch, and dinner parties are the latest diet, the no-fat cheesecake recipe, thigh and hip hatred, and the number of miles they logged on the stair climber.

When you are living in the middle of this, it somehow all seems sane. When you step outside and no longer participate in the obsession, you may feel like walking into the middle of these conversations and yelling, "Get a life!"

Most of the people we identified as unnaturally slim were women. The male counterpart to the unnaturally slim woman might be the unnaturally muscular male. Males easily developed the same obsessions with their bodies and with keeping them not just toned but bulging with masculine muscularity. The diets, supplements, and workouts they were involved in were their top-ics of lunchtime and cocktail hour conversation, just as they were with unnaturally slim women.

Were these people happy? Yes and no. Usually they were "pretty happy with their bodies" except of course for that unruly inch here or there that just would not disappear. They often had many com-plaints about the rest of their lives and how much time it took to maintain their bodies. They also saw themselves as overweight even when they weren't. Were these people healthy? Some were and some were not. Some were what you might call "health freaks" in that they had rules and rituals surrounding their food and what they would and wouldn't eat that *could not* be violated, or it appeared they might lose their minds. Others used cigarettes, liquor, and sex to soothe the stress and pressure they constantly put themselves under. The intensity of their lifestyle was reflected in the tenseness of their brows. I sometimes felt that the precarious state of imbalance they had put their lives in might topple them over the edge at any time.

The very sad part about this is that many of these unnaturally slim people are teaching weight loss programs and fitness classes. Those of us who are in the market to learn how to take better care of our bodies end up seeking guidance from these people and take what they say as the truth. We figure, "They must know what they're talking about—look at their bodies!" I have heard many an aerobics instructor and many a weight loss program instructor say, "I have to teach these classes every day; it forces me to do the program. Otherwise I'd be back to my old fat self." Those comments reveal the underlying truth about what they are teaching. They are teaching a program that cannot be maintained easily and naturally throughout a person's lifetime.

Being Slim Does Not Have to Be an All-Consuming Struggle

We know that a person can become and remain reasonably slim without having to spend every waking moment focused on food and exercise. We also believe that slimness is not just for the rich and famous—those who can afford a cook, a personal trainer, and two or three hours a day off from their job to exercise. Nor does remaining naturally slim for a lifetime require a 25-year food diary! So we continued our search beyond the unnaturally slim. We searched for the masters, the ones who kept slim without an above-average metabolism and without a second thought, those people who had never been on a reducing diet and indeed may have never seen the inside of a health club. We could not advertise for them. They didn't even realize who they were or that they were doing anything special. We kept our eyes open, and one by one as our spotting techniques became more accurate we found these masters. We spotted them in restaurants; we found them in our families and workplaces and at high school reunions. We watched them and talked to them and wrote down their habits.

There was one characteristic that was overwhelmingly present in this group: every single one of them had remained in touch with his or her natural childhood instincts. By remaining in touch with these instincts they stayed very close to optimal body weight all their lives. Staying in touch with their instincts affected not only what and how they ate but also their state of mind. The following information is taken directly from interviews with and questionnaires from naturally slim people:

MW: "I'm 5′6″ and weigh 145 pounds. I stay within one or two pounds of that weight most of the time. I've been on two diets, years ago when I was 10 to 15 pounds above my average. I eat generally around mealtimes and have an occasional snack. I don't like to wait too long to eat, or I get shaky. I don't like buffets—the hot food isn't really hot or the cold food cold."

NC: "I'm 5′7″ and weigh 135 pounds. I like to eat when I first feel hungry; if I wait too long, the hunger becomes strong and then goes away and I lose my appetite. I eat two or three meals and one or two snacks per day. A meal takes me 15 to 30 minutes. I never eat in the car."

GM: "I'm 6′ tall and weigh 155 pounds. I know when to eat by the feeling in my stomach. I eat three meals and two or three snacks a day. I never eat in the car, and a meal usually takes 30 to 45 minutes for me to eat. I'm a picky eater. I like natural foods that are well prepared—not into processed foods. I think about what I eat, but it doesn't occupy a lot of my time. I exercise irregularly, averaging out to three or four hours per week."

VH: "Sometimes I'm a picky eater. I like to eat what appeals to me at the time. I love all foods. Generally I eat three meals and two snacks a day. I exercise informally, but I've enjoyed walking all my life."

JJ: "I'm 5′7″ and wear a size 10 or 12. I dabbled with diets but decided they were too much trouble for too few gains. My weight has been pretty steady all my adult life, with small ups and downs. About eight months ago I started an exercise routine of walking one hour a day. I eat when I'm hungry, and I stop when I'm full."

SS: "I'm 5'2" and weigh 110 pounds. I live alone, and I sometimes eat erratically. Generally I eat lunch and graze the rest of the day. I hate undercooked meat, soggy vegetables, and clumpy rice. I usually do some sort of exercise for 30 minutes five days a week—it could be yoga, tai chi, stretching—I don't belong to a health club. I rarely eat food for comfort, but when I do it's a few chips or chocolate."

LL: "I'm 5'7" tall and weigh around 135 pounds. I've never been on a diet. I eat three meals and three snacks a day and usually spend 20 to 25 minutes at a meal. When my energy level drops, I know I need to eat. I choose small portions at meals. After all, I can eat again soon if I want to."

Just copying the masters' moves will not make you a master. You must also learn how they think and the mental patterns that produce the moves. As you read the next 10 chapters, which reveal the habits of naturally slim people, remember, practicing the moves is important, but *developing the mind-set that supports the moves* is what creates permanent change. The goal is to develop the mind-body-spirit connection that will allow you to make the moves of the masters without a second thought.

Opportunities for Growth

Awareness

- Observe the people around you. Which ones are chronic dieters? Which ones are unnaturally slim? Which ones are naturally slim? How can you tell?

- Watch people you consider slim as they eat. How do they eat? What do they talk about? Are they constantly consumed with conversations about food, diet, exercise, and weight? Can you tell if they are naturally or unnaturally slim?

- If you go to a health club or an exercise class what is the conversation there? Can you pick out the naturally slim people there? Are there any?

Introspection

- How do your thoughts and actions compare with those of naturally slim people? Can you recognize yourself in their profiles, or are they completely foreign to you?

- Is it possible for you to see yourself as normal, with natural instincts?

- What do you really want? If your desire is to be slim at any cost, you may want to rethink your desires. Could you focus on becoming healthy rather than slim?

Old Beliefs to Let Go

You may want to let go of beliefs like these that support being slim by unnatural means:

- Losing weight and keeping it off is hard work.

- I am unable to stay slim for any length of time.

- I am abnormal.

New Beliefs to Embrace

Try these beliefs on for size:

- Reaching my optimal body weight is easy and natural to me.

- I am naturally slim, and I can easily maintain it for life.

- I am normal and natural in every way.

Vividly Imagine

- Start to develop an image of yourself as naturally slim. You will be embellishing this image through all 10 habits. Start to imagine how you look, how you eat, what you feel, what you think and say to yourself.

Patterns for Action

- Interview a friend, neighbor, or relative who is slim. See if you can determine whether she is naturally or unnaturally slim.

- If you can hook up with a naturally slim person, ask him if he would mind validating the information in this book for you.

- Find your own naturally slim master and ask her if you could use her as a mentor. Watch her eat; ask her questions; pick her brain.

Additional Reading

David, Marc. *Nourishing Wisdom*. New York: Bell Tower, 1991.

FOUR

Habit 1: Keep Your Life Priorities Straight

When you step out of the process of dieting and into the process of health, the number of pounds you weigh takes a backseat to making moment-by-moment choices in favor of life.

WHEN WE TALKED to naturally slim people, we asked them what their dreams were, what occupied most of their time and most of their thoughts. The answers they gave had nothing to do with food, weight, or dress size. They mentioned jobs, families, and relationships as well as special causes they were involved in. For the most part they considered themselves active, busy people. They considered good health something that required attention. However, the desire to remain healthy and thin was not the driving force behind their everyday thoughts, feelings, and actions. Most of the naturally slim people we interviewed seemed to operate out of a set of priorities where living a full, productive, satisfying life was at the top, and health maintenance (rather than weight maintenance) was just one small part of it. It is tempting to say, "Well, of course they don't have to worry about their weight. They don't have a weight problem!" Our answer to that is, what if you turned that thought around? They don't have a weight problem because they never put their weight or the shape of their body as their highest life priority.

Life Versus Weight

Meet Sandi. Sandi is an attractive 46-year-old woman who came to our office stating she was 80 pounds over her normal weight. She said she needed some kind of help, but she wasn't sure what. All she knew was that her body disgusted her and that after 25 years of dieting she was the fattest she had ever been. The very first thing we asked Sandi to do was to put her *life* to the mirror test instead of her *body*. When she did, she did not like what she saw. Her daily life was filled with worry, guilt, self-hate, and alternating obsessions and frustrations. She was swamped by feelings that she was never good enough, never had enough time or energy to do all the things she should do. She was always trying to do the right thing but always feeling somehow inadequate. She blamed a lot of these feelings on her body. "If I could just lose some weight," she'd say, "I'd have more energy, I'd be able to do more, and I'd feel better." What Sandi didn't see at first was that many of her overzealous efforts at "doing the right thing," "doing more," and "losing weight" were an attempt to gain approval and acceptance from other people.

You cannot receive from other people what you do not already have for yourself. Sandi needed to start feeling better strictly for herself. The first thing we asked Sandi to do for herself was to declare that she would not diet again. We were not asking her to resign herself to being 80 pounds overweight but to declare that her current obsession with food, calories, exercise, body envy, and body hate was just taking too much time and energy from her life. Sandi—like all of us—deserves better. The process of health does not begin with a fat body and end with a slim one. The process of health is ongoing and three-dimensional. You will develop a slim body as a result of making moment-by-moment choices that are mentally, spiritually, and physically healthy. Starvation, guilt, hate, obsession, low energy, and frustration are a result of a mind-body-spirit system that is out of balance.

When you stop dieting and obsessing about your physical body, you are forced to admit what is really going on in your life. Being overweight is a *symptom* of imbalance. It is not the cause of imbalance. When your size and shape become a nonissue, you free yourself to ponder who you are, what you are doing, what is important to you, and how you are relating to the people around you. How are you relating to your job, to your country, to the universe? What would you like to accomplish in this world before you die?

Like Ebenezer Scrooge, let's take an imaginary walk into the future. You are standing in front of huge iron gates that are the entrance to a cemetery. You walk inside. As you walk over the expanse of soft green grass, you examine the tombstones. One stone that is particularly ornate catches your eye, and you stop to read it:

Here Lies Sarah

Despite Her Genetic Tendencies,
Despite Her Body Type and Her Metabolism,
Against Insurmountable Odds,
She Maintained Her Metropolitan Life Insurance
Ideal Body Weight
Until the Day She Died

Frankly, Sarah, who gives a damn? We are not trying to belittle all the statistics that "prove" being overweight is a health risk. What we are saying is: Don't attack your body and your weight. Instead, attend to your life and your health. Your weight will follow!

What We Really Want Is a Feeling, Not a Dress Size

Take a minute, close your eyes, and imagine a time, maybe just a moment, in your life when you were ecstatic, happy, joyful, serene. Capture that feeling, allow it to flow through your body, and hold it there. Now, think about this carefully: If you could feel that way every moment of every day of your life, would you care what size your body was? No, you wouldn't. Because when most people say that they want to lose weight, what they really want is to *feel* better, to feel happy, joyful, fulfilled, at peace. Perhaps they have bought the media blitz that supports the notion that a slim body is the key to happiness and successful relationships. Perhaps they identify a time in their life when they were happy and remember that they were slim then. They try to recapture those elusive feelings by trying to become slim. Actually what was more likely the case is they were happy and carefree and they maintained a healthy body weight because they felt so good. Many people talk about gradually gaining weight as they get older and talk about slower metabolisms. Maybe instead of a slower metabolism, the burdens they are carrying and the discontent with where their life has taken them keep them just slightly, or a lot, out of touch with their natural instincts, and that is why they begin to put on pounds.

Another elusive feeling that overweight people chase is the high they get on those first few diets that are temporarily successful. They are so elated at having come through the suffering and reached the weight they desired that they feel marvelous and attractive and able to conquer the world. Jane told us the story of one of the first major diets she went on. She had restricted herself to 600 calories a day plus a 100-calorie ice cream bar each night as a treat. She was so elated when her large-boned 5′10″ frame dropped from 180 pounds to 150 pounds that she just kept going! She said it was like a runner's high: "Your body is starving, but your mind is so divorced from any physical feelings that you feel like you could go forever." Well, she kept going until she weighed 130 pounds.

Some people might say that sounds like a fashion model—"What's wrong with that weight?" It might, indeed, be a healthy weight for a fashion model with fine bones and a fast-burning metabolism. But for Jane, a large-boned, muscular woman with a slow-burning metabolism, it was an unhealthy weight, and it was an unmaintainable weight. It's rather like comparing a cantaloupe to a grape. A healthy-sized cantaloupe is a healthy-sized cantaloupe. It is not the size of a grape, nor is it the size of a watermelon. How is it that we can respect and enjoy physical diversity when it comes to fruit but not when it comes to human bodies? A cantaloupe that is the size of a grape is unhealthy. And it will return to its predestined size and shape—just as Jane did. Within one year she was back to 180 pounds.

When people diet themselves down beyond the weight and size that are their genetic and metabolic norm, they find it is impossible to stay there for any length of time. As the weight goes back on, the good feelings disappear and are replaced by guilt, doubt, hate, and despair. People think, sort of as a drug addict or an alcoholic does, perhaps another diet can get me back that feeling, and the self-defeating spiral begins.

At the end of every weight loss/weight gain cycle, each of us has a choice. We can keep on dieting in hopes of reaching that temporary high, or we can step out of the downward spiral knowing that there is more to life than this. Some people make the choice to step out of the spiral after one or two rounds, and some people may take 25 years and 100 rounds. Either way, it is the stepping out that is important, wherever you are in your weight loss history.

When you did the "moment of happiness" exercise at the beginning of the chapter, how long did it take you to come up with that wonderful moment of bliss? How long ago was that moment? When most of our clients do that exercise, we find they go back many years to identify that moment of true joy and peace. If you had to go way back in time to find your blissful moment, that is your first clue that you are not leading a very happy or blissful life now. No matter what you think, this is *not* because you are fat. Your excess body fat is merely a visible, tangible product of your unhappiness that you have chosen to focus on. We are not saying this to make you feel bad. We are saying it so that you might look at yourself and choose to get on the path to growth and change. Through the media, our society supports the notion that weight loss is an important issue to focus your time and money on. But a continued focus on weight loss just allows you to avoid the real issues: you are not as happy as you would like to be, you don't know why, and you don't know what to do about it.

The Possibilities of Life Are Not Determined by Your Weight

Imagine yourself in a world of identical genetic material. Every single person weighs the same as you do, they all have the same facial features, they are the same race, they have the same IQ, and maybe they even have the same amount of money. In this world having excess body fat is normal, acceptable, and expected. In other words, you are now in a world where your weight is a nonissue. Now you are free to be anything you like and to do anything you like. What do you want? What would you like to do that would make you happy? What would bring you happiness and joy? What could you enjoy doing every day for the rest of your life? It is a world of all possibilities. Stay in that world for a while and begin to exercise your rusty imagination. Imagining what you want is the very first step to obtaining it.

Open your eyes. That world is right here, right now!! This is a world of all possibilities. Any limits you have placed on yourself because of your size are only in your mind, and your mind can be changed. Imagining a world where everyone is the same weight forces you to look at yourself and drop all concerns about what other people think. It shows you how you have squelched your own happiness and smothered your dreams because of your need to change your weight before you do anything.

"Well," you might say, "that is very easy for you to say, but I weigh 280 pounds, and I just can't do some of the things I really want to do. I can't get down on the ground and garden; I can't dance; I can't even walk up the steps to the art museum." Maybe right now you can't, but in time, as you step into health and happiness, you will. Remember, health is a process. There are things you can do to support your dreams no matter what size you are. One of our clients, named Lana, is a great example of this process.

Lana the Ballerina

As a child Lana had taken ballet lessons for seven years. She enjoyed it thoroughly and told everyone that she wanted to be a ballerina when she grew up. Lana was a tall, stately girl but very fluid and graceful. She remembers vividly the day she told her very best friend her dream. "I want to be a ballerina when I grow up." Her friend laughed at her out loud. "You can't be a ballerina. You're too big!" At a vulnerable time and age, Lana took that comment to heart. From that time forward she dropped her dream, and soon she even stopped taking ballet lessons. Throughout her adult years she loved to dance at parties but became embarrassed to do so as she gained weight.

Lana's story about her love of dance came out when we were having a discussion about exercise. We asked people to think back to their youth and identify the activities they enjoyed that involved moving their body. Lana of course said ballet. Using psychological kinesiology, which you'll read about in Chapter 17, Lana learned to replace her old belief—that she was too big to dance—with a new belief: "I am a dancer." And she really did believe this. Why wouldn't she—it was true! Three weeks later she decided to go out to the store and buy some ballet shoes. Within eight weeks she had started wearing them around the house. Within three months she had called several ballet studios but decided to continue, for the moment, to confine her dancing to the house when she was alone. However, within a little more than a year she had signed up to take lessons one night a week. If she had just used willpower and gone out and *made* herself sign up for lessons before she was ready, she probably would have quit and never gone back. It was because she gave herself a belief that supported dancing, and she gave herself time to integrate that belief into action, that she is now able to partially live out her dream and improve her health at the same time.

Who are you? What do you really want? What is really important to you? What are your life priorities? When you list your life priorities, stop and look at a day, a week, or a month. Is the majority of what you think and do spent on your highest priorities? If your top priority is raising healthy children or saving the rain forest, is your time spent supporting that priority? Or do you spend most of your time in guilt and worry about your body, the results of your current diet, and the amount of fat grams in one bread versus another? Understanding the principles of nutrition is important to good health, but look at the time you spend on it—is it appropriate?

Who Are You, Anyway?

Who am I? is a critical question to ask yourself when determining your life priorities. Ask yourself this question and look closely at your answers. When you ask yourself, "Who am I?" do you refer to yourself as a wife, husband, mother, father, girlfriend, sister, son, lover? Most people describe themselves in relation to other people. The second most common way people describe themselves is in terms of what they do—"I'm a banker, plumber, housewife, lawyer." Or, they may say, "I'm a tall blond German," referring to their physical characteristics and their heritage. If we were all just physical bodies, genetic tendencies, and jobs, then in that fantasy world where everyone looked the same and had the same job, people would be clones—they would think and act exactly alike. But they don't think and act alike. Are identical twins the same people? Of course not. They are individuals. They don't think or act exactly alike, they don't imagine things in the same way, and they don't react to any given situation in the same way.

Each of us has a part that is unique regardless of any other physical trappings. I call this the *spirit*. Others call it the *true self* or the *higher self*, and some call it the *essence* or the *life force*. Whatever you call it, very few people deny that it takes something besides blood, bone, and brain to make a human being who she or he is. You are a spirit that lives in a body and has a mind. You have unique talents and abilities as well as unique life experiences that make you the living, thinking, loving person who you are. You have a purpose on this earth that is uniquely yours, and your quest to know your true self and find your purpose in life will do more for your physical body than any weight loss diet will ever do.

Once you know and love that spirit part of you and straighten out the thoughts and beliefs in your mind so that they support that spirit self, a naturally healthy physical body will follow. This is a process, a growing process. It will take time. But healthy growth usually does. When a cell grows uncontrollably fast, they call it cancer! True and lasting change takes place from the inside out. Changing what you eat or how you exercise without ever changing the thoughts and beliefs and unawareness that brought you to be fat will never produce a pleasurable lasting change. The first step is to begin to recognize that you are more than a body, that you are a unique spirit with a purpose here that no one else can fill. Look at your life and begin to rearrange those priorities so that your time is spent on what is important to you. It is OK if loving yourself and being happy are a priority in your life. Remember, you cannot give away what you do not have. Any thoughts of loving and service to others will only flow freely from you when you love and serve your true self.

Opportunities for Growth

Awareness

- Close your eyes and recall a moment in time when you felt happy, blissful, fulfilled. Allow that feeling to penetrate every fiber of your body. Sit with this feeling of bliss and enjoy it. Once you have the feeling strongly anchored in your body, drop the image you were thinking of and just hold the feeling. Practice this when you are watching a sunrise or sunset. Feel that pleasant, all-is-right-with-the-world feeling. Know that you can have that feeling whenever you want.

Introspection

- Imagine you live in a world where weight is not an issue for you or anyone else. Imagine that everyone is over-weight and that that is the norm. In a world of all possibilities, with your weight a nonissue, what do you really want out of life?

- Ask yourself, "Who am I? Am I able to accept that I am more than my body? That I am more than my job? That I am more than a relative to someone else?" Begin to realize that you have worth and value just because you are you.

- What are your life priorities other than changing your body size? List them and rank them if you want. Now take a day and notice how much thought and energy you put into each of those priorities. Is it balanced? Or is your mind cluttered with unrelated issues that keep you from what means the most to you?

Old Beliefs to Let Go

Here are some very self-defeating things you say to yourself that support exactly what you don't want:

- I'm too old to change.

- Life is passing me by.

- When I lose some weight, I'll _____. (Fill in the blank.)

- I'll never get to do what I really want to do.

- I can't do _____; that's impossible. (Fill in the blank.)

New Beliefs to Embrace

- The possibilities in my life are unlimited.

- I am ready, willing, and able to live my dreams now.

- Whatever I vividly imagine and sincerely believe will happen in my life.

Vividly Imagine

- Select one of your life priorities that has nothing to do with your weight. Now imagine yourself, step by step, spending time and doing exactly what you have always wanted to do in that area of your life.

Patterns for Action

- Pick one small, first step from your vivid image and carry through with it. Remember Lana, the ballerina. Pick steps that are small enough that you can experience success every step of the way.

Additional Reading

Chopra, Deepak, M.D. *Seven Spiritual Laws of Success.* San Rafael: Amber-Allen Publishing and New World Library, 1993.

Covey, Stephen. *The 7 Habits of Highly Effective People.* New York: Fireside Press, 1990.

Simon, Sidney, Dr. *In Search of Values: 31 Strategies for Finding Out What Really Matters Most to You.* New York: Warner, 1993.

Habit 2: Love Yourself . . . Body, Mind, and Spirit

Love is the most powerful resource we have.
We were all born with an unlimited supply of
unconditional self-love within us. Yet many
people spend their entire lives searching for that
love somewhere else.

THE MAJORITY OF the naturally slim people we interviewed liked themselves. They had a high degree of self-esteem or self-love. Naturally slim people do not love themselves because they are slim; they love themselves for who they are. Waiting to like yourself until you become a certain size will never allow you to become naturally slim. It takes an unconditional love of self to be kind, loving, patient, and supportive to yourself during the natural weight loss process. It takes a love of self to give yourself the time you need to read this book, do the exercises, eat differently, and incorporate healthy habits into your life. You cannot afford to wait until you become slim to like yourself. You've been doing that for years, and what has it gotten you? Becoming naturally slim is dependent on developing a healthy level of self-love.

True Love Is Unconditional

Overweight people often withhold love from themselves, thinking that this will somehow motivate them to stay on their latest diet or exercise regime. This is completely erroneous. Love, not the withholding of love, motivates us toward health. Loving yourself only if you perform a certain way or look a certain way is called *conditional love.* This is not really love at all. True love is unconditional; I love you right or wrong, fat or thin, rich or poor, healthy or unhealthy. Loving yourself or someone else only if certain conditions are met says that *what we do* is more important than *who we are.*

Think about an infant or a young child, so ready to accept the world without conditions, eager to love people for who they are without regard to size or shape or color. A two-year-old jumps into the lap of his dying grandfather and hugs him because he's Grandpa. The child doesn't care if Grandpa is thin and sallow and bald from chemotherapy. The love is unconditional. The love is for the spirit of who Grandpa is, not Grandpa's body. Unconditional self-love is ours by nature. Self-hate and conditional love are learned. Be eager to unlearn them!

The word *love* is used so often these days its power as a source of energy for our spirit is often lost. We "love" a new hairstyle, we "love" a certain book, and we just "loved" our last vacation. Words such as *admire* and *like* could easily be used and give a much more accurate portrayal of the depth of feelings involved.

Don't let overuse of the word cause you to be numb to the true power of love. Love is the most powerful resource we have within us. We were all born with it. Yet, if we believe the messages generated by both visual and print media, love can be found only outside ourselves and usually with a person of the opposite sex. Mesmerized by some convoluted idea of romantic love, millions of people spend their lives searching for love in all the wrong places. They search for that special someone who will love them, that someone who will fill the emptiness inside. What they often don't understand is that they are looking for someone else to give them what they cannot give themselves. The truth is, if we fill that emptiness by loving ourselves, the desperate need for a special someone else goes away and we become much more peaceful, lovable people.

Look in the Mirror and
Say the Words

We would like you to consider love in the purest sense of the word and then think about it in terms of yourself, not someone else. Look up the word *love* in a dictionary. To love is to have a strong liking for, to cherish, to adore, to respect, to hold in high esteem, to have reverence for. The word *love*, like a seed, is filled with potential. As you read and say its meanings over and over, it grows in strength and wisdom that touches the heart. Can you take each one of these synonyms for love and say them about yourself? Look into your own eyes, the windows to your soul, in a mirror and say, "I cherish myself." "I respect myself." "I hold myself in high esteem." "I love myself." Loving yourself is not a narcissistic, selfish endeavor. It is a kind, generous, powerful thing to do. For only when you unconditionally love and accept yourself in spirit, mind, and body can love begin to overflow into other areas of your life. This includes loving yourself enough to take the time to become healthy and naturally slim instead of going on another diet. Loving yourself enough to take the time to read this book and do the exercises. Loving yourself enough to want to get to know yourself and your physical instincts of hunger and satiety. Loving yourself enough to learn how to change beliefs that are limiting your health and your life. Loving yourself enough to stop dieting because it is hurtful and you do not hurt someone you love.

If you have tried the mirror exercise in the last paragraph you may have found out how little you really love yourself at this moment. Perhaps a little voice kept saying, "No way," or perhaps you had to grit your teeth and set your jaw to say it, or perhaps doing this exercise brought you to tears. Don't be afraid of tears. They may be the first honest emotions you've allowed yourself to release in a very long time. The tears are part of your grief for the many years you abandoned your true self, the years you stayed away from mirrors and love so that you wouldn't have to feel the pain. There is no need for guilt about this. You did the best you knew how to do at the time. But now you know more and you are open to learning a different perspective on life, yourself, food, and your body. Now you can proceed differently if you choose. Loving yourself in body, mind, and spirit is not something that will happen overnight.

Developing a Loving Relationship with Yourself Takes Time

Rekindling the loving relationship that you had with yourself when you were born takes time, just like rekindling a relationship with an old friend. There are stages you will go through. First, you need to spend time with yourself. Become better acquainted with who you are and what makes you tick. When was the last time you sat by yourself, alone, and without a television, radio, or telephone turned on? Have you stopped and listened to what kinds of thoughts go through your head? Can you sit still with a flower in your hand and just enjoy the pure beauty of its nature? What is your nature? What do you perceive as beautiful? Fun? Important? Unimportant? Do worries about the future and regrets about the past occupy your mind frequently? Do you enjoy what you are doing in your life day to day? These are just a few of the questions you might ask yourself in order to get to know yourself better. Using the introspection exercises in this book will also introduce you to parts of yourself. You can also learn about your-self by noticing your reactions to the people around you. What are your reactions and where do they come from?

From this you can begin to develop a friendship with your-self. However, as the friendship becomes more intimate, you may also become aware of things you don't like about yourself. Don't abandon the relationship because of these things and don't go on a wild crusade to change them all at once. Decide to accept yourself with all of your frailties. Decide to accept yourself, even if you do not change a thing. Remember, true love is unconditional. Say to yourself, especially to the part of yourself you may disapprove of, "I accept you exactly the way you are. I may prefer that you be different, and I may in the future decide to change some things about you, but right this moment I accept you exactly as you are." Acquaintance, friendship, intimacy, and acceptance form a foundation for not just liking yourself but loving yourself.

Love Your Spirit

A loving relationship with yourself means loving your spirit, your mind, and your body in balance—not choosing one or the other as your life focus but choosing all three simultaneously and equally. We are going to guess, however, that most of you are out of balance and may have been so for decades. You may have spent the majority of your days, year after year, working on or lamenting your physical body. Therefore, we are going to ask you to decrease the time you spend working on your physical body and invest that time in loving your spirit and your mind. We usually suggest that you begin with your spirit. As you get to know your spirit self, your essence, your true self, you will rapidly come to the conclusion "What's not to love?" Your spirit self *is* love. It is the part of you, buried under years of mental programming, that is loving, deserving, willing, giving, joyous, blissful, and carefree. It is the light that is shining through your life when everything feels right, when you are flowing, at peace and happy. The fact that those times may be few and far between right now does not mean that they have to remain that way or that your spirit is dead.

Your spirit cannot die. However, you can spend a lifetime not ever knowing it or allowing it to influence the way you think and act. Ponder the questions we asked in Chapter 4 when you looked at your life priorities. Who are you really? Not what do you do for a living or who your ancestors were, but *who* are you? What are the unique qualities of the spirit that you bring into the world? What are your strengths? What do you consider your weaknesses? It's possible that what you consider a weakness in yourself may indeed be your gift to the world.

Take for instance a client of ours named Darcy. As Darcy was working on a new relationship with herself, she pondered the fact that she had spent many years as vice president or co-chair of a wide variety of organizations. In her own words, she ". . . spent many years in positions where I played second fiddle to some very powerful, dynamic women." Darcy knew that she had the leadership skills to be in the top job, but somehow she never was. At first she saw this as some sort of character defect such as a lack of motivation. She thought she was doing it to dodge responsibility. "In fact," she said, "when I was working as a nurse, people would say, 'You're so bright. Why didn't you become a doctor?' I would laugh and tell them I didn't want *that* much responsibility." The truth was, she loved being a nurse and being a doctor held no interest for her. Did that mean she had a character defect? It was not until Darcy was on her journey to know and love herself that she discovered that the very qualities she was bemoaning as defects were her greatest strengths and the key to her life's purpose. Darcy is a catalyst for dynamic action. She is able to be in the middle of any situation and see the whole picture, put things in perspective. She's a spark for creative solutions that might not have been seen if she had not been present. Yes, she's a "middleman." She is not interested in position or power.

Now Darcy is able to accept and love herself for who she is rather than thinking she should be something "better." *Better* implies a value judgment. Is being president "better" than being vice president? Is being an apple "better" than being an orange? Begin to look at yourself without judgment. Find that spark, that strength that is uniquely yours. Maybe it's your sense of humor; maybe it's your compassion; maybe it's even something you thought was a weakness. Whatever those qualities, they are sure to be the ones that bring out the loving, deserving, willing, joyous core within you that is your spirit. Let that part of you guide your thoughts and actions and it will never let you down.

Deep down we all want to feel better about ourselves. Our mistake has been to attach those good feelings to the shape of our physical body. When we begin to recognize our unique spiritual qualities and love ourselves for those, it is easy to feel better about ourselves—one step at a time.

Love Your Mind

It has been said that whatever you vividly imagine, fervently desire, believe with all your heart, and act on with energy and enthusiasm must come to pass. The mind is not simply a brain. It is much, much more. It is intelligence and memory far more powerful than any computer whiz could ever dream of, and its potential for creative thought is unlimited. Memories and message-carrying proteins called *neurotransmitters* are not limited to the confines of the brain but can be found in every cell of the body. We are, quite literally, what we think! As infants and young children we soak up experiences like a sponge. Though our brains may be hardwired through genetics when we are born, there are still billions upon billions of neuronal paths and patterns that are determined by life experiences—the look of love in a father's eye, the startling sound of a doorbell, the discomfort of a wet diaper. Each moment of our lives brings input to our conscious and subconscious mind. Experiences that are repeated often become the beliefs through which we view the world. If almost every time your brother walks into the living room he gives you a whack on the head, the connection is soon made that seeing your brother means pain. In time you will cringe and close your eyes and your heart will pound whenever you see your brother coming, whether he hits you or not. We formulate our beliefs, thoughts, and ultimately our actions from the experiences in our lives.

If a picture is worth a thousand words, then a mental image is worth at least a million. We can imagine a large black hairy spider so vividly that our flesh crawls with goose bumps and we break out into a cold sweat. We can visualize a setting so peaceful that we reduce our heart rate by 40 percent. We can react with such intensity to the events in our lives that we create ulcers in our own stomach! Our minds can make mountains out of molehills or molehills out of mountains—and what is even neater is that we can *choose* which we want to do! Understand and appreciate the power of your mind. Realize that it is possible that the beliefs you have developed about yourself and the ways in which you think can literally keep you fat. Also realize that the same power can create new beliefs and thoughts that help you to let go of your fat. Excess fat is not just a physical thing. It is a mental thing and a spiritual thing as well.

The goose bumps, the sweating, the reduction in heart rate, and the ulcers are all evidence that you have the power to manifest physical events just by thinking about them. Imagine what you could accomplish if you harnessed that power to work in favor of your own health and happiness. Your mind is the intermediary between your spirit self and your physical self. The only thing standing in the way of your true spiritual nature's (happiness, health, wisdom, etc.) being manifested in your physical body is the state of your mind. Love your mind by appreciating its power and then using it in your favor.

Start to become aware of your thoughts and reactions in all kinds of situations. Does what you're thinking make you feel good? Happy? Loving? Peaceful? All those spiritual qualities that can make life grand? If not, consider changing the way you think. Become aware of how you think and react, and if you don't like what you discover, acknowledge that you have the power to *change* your thoughts, to *change* your reactions, and let yourself make that change. You may have spent years cluttering up your mind with negative, limiting thoughts: "I'm too old." "That's just the way I am." "My job is high stress; I can't help it." "I am so angry I feel like I could rip him apart." "I'm fat and unattractive." "I'll never be healthy." And so forth. Consider now what might happen if you thought differently.

If chronic stress and anger can eat holes in your stomach, can chronic peace and harmony heal them? The answer to this question is yes! You can change your physical health, including the amount of excess body weight you are carrying around, by changing the state of your mind. In fact, changing the way you think is mandatory to continue making behavior changes that are permanent. A mind that is open and positive and that allows your spirit to shine through into your life is a mind that is ready to develop natural, loving eating and exercise habits. It is a mind that will allow your true, naturally slim nature to emerge.

Details concerning techniques that are useful in changing the way you think will be provided in subsequent chapters. We also encourage you to read some of the books in the resource list at the end of this chapter.

Love Your Body

Until now, you may have spent most of your life focusing solely on your body—the physical part of who you are. Now is the time to put this in third place in your areas of focus, behind developing your spirit and your mind. This does not mean to ignore your body until you get the other parts straightened out. All three are important and interdependent. However, allowing your *spirit* to be the driving force in your life and keeping your state of *mind* supportive of that force will have more impact on your physical health than any food or exercise plan you can ever imagine. From a loving spirit and a loving mind will flow a love for your body, no matter what shape it is. A loving spirit and a loving mind also facilitate dissolving your old relationship with your body and developing a new one. A new relationship with your body can be approached in the same manner in which you approach any relationship: acquaintance, friendship, intimacy, acceptance, and love. Even if acceptance is as far as you get in your relationship with your body, you'll be eons away from the body hate that you once felt.

We encourage you to use mirror work as you come to know your body. Stand in front of a mirror, look directly into your own eyes, and state the positive beliefs you want to have about yourself. No matter what size it is, see your body as a wonderfully functioning machine. Billions of reactions are taking place at any given time, providing life to each cell, detoxifying poisons, building muscles, healing wounds—the miracles are endless. Begin to see your body as a friend and not as an enemy. It is the one and only physical house you have been given for that indomitable spirit of yours. You will want it to be healthy so you can live your life to its fullest potential. Limb by limb, organ by organ, understand the miracle that your body is. Appreciate it for how it has gotten you through your life so far in spite of whatever dieting or exercise abuse you've subjected it to!

When our clients first begin mirror work, often they can only look at their eyes or hair and remain positive. Later they are able to add their mouth or their ears and say something loving about them. We ask our clients not to move on to another body part until they can truly say they accept and appreciate the one they are looking at. Believe it or not, you can look in the mirror and be OK with wrinkles, moles, and double chins. Don't judge your face or body against some arbitrary standard of beauty. Understand that your body is the shape it is because of the past—the way you used to think, the way you used to act, the way you used to eat and exercise. Accept that you did the best that you could at the time and look to a future of health.

If you had a child with a physical problem, would you refuse to look at him, touch him, or buy him nice clothes? Of course not, because you love that child and accept him just as he is. That is the least you can do for yourself. Getting acquainted with the loose flab on your upper arms or the rolls on your belly may be challenging. But it is very helpful in developing a healthy attitude about yourself. Hate is very unsuccessful as a motivator. Before I ever lost a pound I was able to look at myself naked in a mirror and feel OK with my body, to appreciate that it had many, many pounds of excess fat. I also appreciated that I had gained that fat through ignorance and self-hate, and I acknowledged that that was history. I knew I was on my way to renewed health and vigor; that dwelling on the body of my past was not helpful; that envisioning my future body *was*.

The greatest support you can give yourself while you are making changes in your life is love—unconditional love for who you are right now, without guilt about the past, worry about the future, or judgment in the present.

Opportunities for Growth

Awareness

- Note the physical effects you can create in your own body by vividly imagining a huge hairy spider crawling up your leg, or squeezing the sour juice of a fresh-cut lemon onto your tongue. Watch a scary movie and feel the goose bumps and the rapid heart rate as you become totally immersed in the vivid experience. Think of your own examples of your mind causing a physical reaction in your body.

- Become aware of who you are, body, mind, and spirit, by spending some time with the person you need to love most, yourself. Talk to yourself, write to yourself, do something you have always wanted to do. Try spending some quiet time in nature. It gives you a feeling of connectedness, and trees are extremely good listeners!

- Begin to look at yourself in the mirror. Remember there is no good or bad way to look; there is just what is. Accept your body as a creation of your life's experiences and know that it will evolve as new experiences are incorporated into your life. Start small and slow, take your time, forgive yourself for the hate and disparaging remarks you have loaded on yourself. You created this body, large or small, and it is the only one you have. Promise to take care of it more lovingly in the future. Give yourself a hug.

Please note: If this or any other exercise brings you to tears, don't be frightened. Be glad—it means you have hit a truth that your spirit wants you to recognize. Just stop what you're doing, go someplace comfortable, and cry it out. At the end of your tears, keep your mind open for an idea or an insight that might occur to you.

Introspection

- Think about what makes you a unique person with something to give the world. What qualities do you have that make you a dynamic, lovable human being? What aspects of yourself do you consider weaknesses? Could they really be strengths in disguise? Do you compare your qualities against other people's to decide whether yours "measure up" or are "worthwhile"?

Old Beliefs to Let Go

- I'm ugly and fat.

- I hate my _____ (body, hips, thighs, arms, face, other).

- I'm worthless.

- Nobody loves me.

New Beliefs to Embrace

- I accept myself and my body.

- I appreciate my body; therefore I care for it with love.

- I am a spirit being, and my body is the house I live in.

- I am a person of worth and value, and I hold myself in high esteem.

Vividly Imagine

- Imagine yourself and all your positive spiritual qualities. If you erased every self-limiting thought from your mind right now, where would you be? What would you be doing? What would you look like?

Patterns for Action

- Choose one aspect of yourself that you really like and flaunt it, play with it, learn how good it feels to like yourself. If you're a good dancer, turn on some music and dance. If you have beautiful eyes, try a new eye shadow. If you sing; join a choir or just belt one out in the shower.

- Look at your body and pick one aspect that you like about your physical self. Tell yourself each day how much you like and appreciate your _____ (eyes, hair, smile, etc.). Add a new body part every week or two, including your thighs, hips, and stomach. Make peace with your body, accept it, and appreciate it just the way it is.

Additional Reading

Hay, Louise. *You Can Heal Your Life.* Santa Monica: Hay House, 1984.

Hirschmann, Jane, and Carol Munter. *When Women Stop Hating Their Bodies.* New York: Fawcett Columbine, 1995.

Johnson, Carol. *Self-Esteem Comes in All Sizes.* New York: Doubleday, 1995.

Moyers, Bill. *Healing and the Mind.* New York: Doubleday, 1993.

Rodin, Judith, Ph.D. *Body Traps.* New York: William Morrow and Company, Inc., 1992.

Roth, Geneen. *Feeding the Hungry Heart.* Indianapolis: Bobbs-Merrill, 1982.

Roth, Geneen. *When Food Is Love.* New York: Plume, 1992.

Seigel, Bernie, M.D. *Love, Medicine and Miracles.* New York: Harper and Row, 1986.

Six

Habit 3: Free Yourself from Judgment and Guilt

Day after day we judge ourselves as good or bad based on what we are eating or how we look. If we release ourselves from the tyranny of judgment, guilt, and worry, we can free up enormous amounts of time and energy to be used in more positive ways.

NATURALLY SLIM PEOPLE can be as judgmental as the rest of us about the weather, the local football team, or the state of our government. However, they are not judgmental when it comes to food. To them, food is food. They eat just about anything they like in moderation. They have personal likes and dislikes, and they may avoid certain foods because they are not very healthy, but only a few of the naturally slim people we interviewed labeled certain foods as "good" or "bad." Even if they did label them, that did not mean they never ate them; it meant they rarely ate them, usually for health reasons. In contrast, chronic dieters and unnaturally slim people consider many foods "bad" or "forbidden." Usually labeling foods "good" or "bad" is intended to promote healthy eating, which is laudable. However, two major problems arise when we label foods this way.

One problem occurs when people begin to associate their "goodness" or "badness" as a person with their choices of "good" or "bad" foods. A second problem occurs when people become rigid, deciding they will *never* eat certain foods, because they are "bad." Often these "bad" foods are foods that have brought them much pleasure over the years. Not being able to eat them anymore triggers feelings of deprivation. It has been said that whatever we are deprived of we often become obsessed by, so when the "I never eat that" people finally break down and "cheat," they don't eat just one or two pieces of the forbidden food but binge uncontrollably. This binge is usually followed by an overwhelming sense of failure and guilt that is way out of proportion to the "crime."

Needing to Be Right Limits Our Ability to Grow

Most of us invest huge amounts of time and energy into being right. We want to do the right thing, be in the right place at the right time, be seen with the right people, wear the right clothes, eat the right foods, and of course, be the right weight for our height. We engage in many an argument defending what we think is right, whether it has to do with the current political state of our country or the brand of disposable diapers we use for our babies.

Personally, I used cloth diapers for my children because I felt it was better for the environment. If I were to make that statement to a person who was using disposable diapers, it would probably trigger feelings of guilt and anger. The thought pattern might run something like this: "Maybe she's *right*. Maybe I *should* use cloth diapers." "I feel *bad* that I may be contaminating the environment, but cloth diapers are such a pain." "I suppose it *shouldn't* matter if it's a pain if it's the *right* thing to do." "Who does she think she is anyway with that 'holier than thou' attitude?" "I wish she and her environmental friends would just drop dead!" My my my, what a stew of guilt and anger we can think ourselves into. If we admit that someone else is "right," that makes us "wrong." By connecting our sense of self-worth with the rightness of our opinions, we feel threatened down to our core if we are challenged. The truth is, there is not one universally right or wrong way to do anything, whether it's raising children or losing weight.

Releasing ourselves from the self-imposed tyranny of always needing to know and do what is "right" can be extremely liberating. We are not meant to be slaves to standards of rightness, regardless of whether we created the standards or adopted them from someone else. We are meant to live a life of *awareness* and *choice*. A life that flows and bends like a river, sometimes forging a new path, sometimes following an old one; sometimes running headlong into rocks and bouncing up in the air without a thought of where the "right" place is to land. A life that is filled with loving, learning, growing, and having fun. A life of physical, mental, and spiritual fulfillment.

Guilt and Judgment Undermine Our Progress Toward Health

We all have the same raw material, the same potential as Albert Einstein or Amelia Earhart. So with unlimited potential, healthy natural instincts, and the freedom to choose, how do we manifest the slim healthy body we were born to have? That is what these 10 habits are all about. You can choose to set your life priorities straight, you can choose to love yourself, and you can choose to trade judgment and guilt for curiosity and awareness, especially when it comes to your body and your eating habits.

Your physical body right now is a manifestation of all the experiences you have had since you were an infant. Knowing that you may have become fat to protect yourself is a valuable insight when taken in the spirit of curiosity and awareness. However, pronouncing judgment on what you did as "bad" and feeling guilty because you did it is *not* valuable. Guilt is an unhealthy state of mind that undermines, rather than supports, the process of health. Feeling guilty does not make you a better person, nor does it change what has already happened. If it feels like guilt, get rid of it.

Now, mind you, we did *not* say you were "wrong" or "bad" for feeling guilty. Don't judge your feelings. Feelings are not right or wrong; they just are. In fact, feelings, positive or negative, are helpful messengers that ask us to pay attention to the state of our mind and our spirit. Identify your feeling; call it by name. Then step out of the feeling and decide if you want to continue to feel that way. Do you really enjoy this feeling of guilt? If not, learn from it. Find out what thoughts you were thinking that made you feel that way. Catch yourself the next time your thoughts move in that direction—maybe you can stop the guilt before it starts. Remember, you cannot feel guilt unless you are reliving the past. The place that you want to be for positive dynamic change is in the present moment.

Worry Is Guilt's First Cousin

Just as guilt involves remorseful feelings about the past, worry involves anxious feelings about the future. Looking forward in anxiety, concerned about whether you will be able to lose a certain amount of weight by Christmas or summer vacation is called *worrying*. Worry, like guilt, is a nonproductive use of thoughts. Have you ever accomplished anything with the energy of worry? Think about it: worrying about whether your jeans will fit, worrying about whether it will rain, worrying about whether your child will be hit by a car. What has it done? Worrying does not affect the outcome of an event. The truth is, when you put on the jeans, either they will fit or they won't; either you will take them off or you won't; and either you will wear something different or you won't. You are not "good" or "bad" because they don't fit. Feeling guilty because you gained weight and can't fit into your jeans will not make them fit any differently. Remember that where you want to be for positive growth and change is in the present moment, with awareness and curiosity. If you are worrying, you are in the future and your thought energy is wasted on nongrowth. If you are feeling guilty, you are in the past and your thought energy is wasted on nongrowth. Holy Toledo! No wonder we are all so tired all the time. If we could tap into all the energy spent in this world on guilt and worry, we could probably eliminate the need for nuclear power plants!

If you become aware that you are immersed in judgment, guilt, or worry, remember that you are not "bad" because you are there. Decide if you are enjoying yourself, and if you aren't, learn from the experience and move on. Take judgment out of your decisions. Many of these judgments are based on a set of beliefs and values handed to you by your parents and the world you grew up in. Now, as an adult, you need to reevaluate those beliefs and trade them in for new ones if they don't provide a foundation for health and happiness. You are not bound forever to "clean your plate" and "eat your vegetables before you can have dessert." Nor do you have to be a slave to unrealistic standards of beauty that are presented by the media.

When you establish a sense of love and respect for who you are in body, mind, and spirit, you can stop judging yourself so harshly. At this time in your life, food, weight, and body issues have sent you to this book for help and information. Removing judgment, guilt, and worry about what you eat and how you look is a place to start. When you release these nonproductive attitudes, you free up an enormous amount of thought energy that can be used to assimilate new naturally slim habits into your life.

There Are No "Good" or "Bad" Foods

As I typed this heading, I could hear the gasps of millions of Americans. In their heads they were saying, "Everyone knows that fat and sugar are bad." "Also red meat and rich desserts are bad." "Mashed potatoes are OK, but gravy is really bad." The list goes on and on. What's on your list of bad foods? Who created that list? How do you feel when you pass up a dessert based on the belief that it is bad? I'll bet that you feel deprived. What happens when you feel deprived? The single slice of chocolate cake you righteously passed up at dinner sits in the refrigerator and calls your name. Late in the evening you may consume not only the dessert you passed up but several others besides.

Food is food. Some food is more nutrient dense than others. Some food provides higher-quality and longer-lasting energy than others. Some foods tend to leave residues in your blood vessels and contribute to ill health. Some foods have very low fuel quality for your body, but they were made by your mom and they feed your soul. But food is not "good" or "bad," and more important, *you* are not "good" or "bad" because you ate or didn't eat a particular food!

Through the process of health that you are learning you will develop an awareness of the qualities of various foods. As you come to trust your body and its natural instincts toward health, you will prefer health-supporting foods. The first step in the process of choosing to eat healthy foods for life is to be aware of when, where, what, and how much you are eating and why. Put a sign up in your kitchen: "I am awake and aware when I eat." Make notes in your calendar or journal: "Friday, 10:30 P.M., three bowls of chocolate chip ice cream. I was not at all hungry; I just was tired and exhausted and numb." Remember, *no guilt!* Absolutely every eating experience is a learning experience. Instead of feeling guilty about having eaten ice cream to comfort yourself, know that you were taking care of yourself the best way you knew how. You are gathering up learning experiences that will assist you in making healthy changes.

Look at all the things you could learn from that one experience: (1) Sometimes you need comfort. (2) Feeling numb means you're not feeling at all. (3) Friday night is a vulnerable time for you. (4) You're awfully tired, and maybe you need more sleep. (5) Why chocolate chip ice cream? Is it the chocolate you like or the coldness or the creaminess? If you can remain curious and aware during your eating experiences instead of judgmental and guilt-ridden, each experience, whether a binge or a snack, can contribute to your progress toward health.

Preferences for healthy foods are developed over time. Abruptly replacing your Friday night chocolate chip ice cream with celery sticks will not work. Most of the reasons you're eating that chocolate chip ice cream have nothing to do with your stomach and everything to do with your mind. I don't know about you, but I have very few comfort associations with celery sticks. In fact, they remind me of many dreadful diets I've been on. This is why diets have little success. They do not help you understand and address the psychological associations that you have with foods. You will be able to reduce your Friday night ice cream from three bowls to one, or you may give it up altogether, when you begin to meet your comfort needs on a regular basis in other, healthier ways.

There Are No "Good" or "Bad" Body Sizes

Is a size-8 person "good" and a size-28 person "bad"? I know people of both sizes, and believe me, who they truly are as people is unrelated to their size. We, the American public, are very judgmental of people who are overweight. We have attached judgments of laziness, weak-willedness, sloppiness, jolliness, lack of caring, and more to the amount of fat a person has stored on his or her body. In a research study, children five and six years old were shown pictures of people with various physical differences. One person was on crutches, one person was blind, one was in a wheelchair, and one was obese. When asked which person they would least like to be, 90 percent of the children said they would least like to be the fat person. Our judgments associated with body size are reaching children at a very early age. We now have average-sized seven- and eight-year-old girls going on "diets" and thinking they are fat, many of them using their mothers as role models.

The amount of fat a person has stored on his or her body is merely a result of genetics and past relationships with food. It gives us no information about the qualities of that person. I laugh especially hard when people refer to those who are overweight as being "weak-willed." Some of the strongest-willed persons I know are those who have steadfastly returned to dieting over and over again and gained weight in spite of their diligence. Often these people are trying to reach a weight that is totally unrealistic for their body type and metabolism. Personally, I was 5′10″ tall, weighed 158 pounds, and wore a size 14 before I started dieting. I was not overweight for my height and body type. However, I thought I was fat and began dieting. Twenty-five years and 50 diets later I was 5′10″ and 240 pounds. Was I a bad person? No, but I sure felt bad. The bad feelings were a direct result of accepting other people's judgments of me as true. I took those judgments into my heart, and I was a very sad and angry person.

You Can Never Win or Lose; You Can Only Win or Learn

We determined earlier that guilt and worry consume time and energy with absolutely no positive result. In fact, guilt and worry have a negative impact on our lives not only by occupying time in nongrowth activity but also by compromising our feelings of self-worth and impinging on the joy we are meant to experience. Feeling guilty is our judgment of ourselves and our actions. We judge them against an arbitrary standard of what is good or right—what "should" be. Whenever you hear yourself using the word *should*, catch yourself and know that you are in a spiral of guilt, self-recrimination, and ultimate bad feelings. Rethink the situation you are in without judgment and see how you can intercept the judgmental thought patterns that may lead you to be unhappy. Remember there is no good or bad in the journey to becoming naturally slim. There is no win or lose. There is only win or learn. Adopt the attitude in every situation you are in that you have a preference for the way it turns out, but if it doesn't turn out that way you will learn a valuable lesson. You are either blooming or growing. Either way you can't lose!

Dining Without Judgment

Let's take a look at a dining experience from two perspectives: first, the dieter who is still steeped in judgment and guilt, and second, the naturally slim person who believes in the win/learn philosophy. Imagine that you are sitting in a restaurant. You have completed dinner and you are more than comfortably full; in fact, you have eaten way more than you intended. The dessert cart is brought to the table, and it includes your all-time favorite, flourless chocolate cake. Here is the conversation that occurs in millions of diet heads across America every Friday and Saturday night: "Oh, wow! My favorite!" (joy, elation) "Oh, no, I don't have any room. I'm stuffed." (disappointment) "I really want that cake, and I haven't had it in months." (desire driven by deprivation) "I really shouldn't get dessert." (guilt) "I'm too fat already." (judgment and self-flagellation) "But I really want it, and who knows when I'll have an opportunity to have it again?" (desire, obsession driven by deprivation in the past and a plan to continue the deprivation into the future) "I'll take the cake!" (joy) The cake is usually eaten fairly rapidly, as if someone might take it away; then the thoughts begin again: "Why did I do that? I have no willpower. I'm never going to lose any weight." (guilt, worry, self-recrimination, punishment) The cake was, to say the least, not very satisfying under these circumstances.

Here's the same scenario, only from the perspective of a person with a naturally slim win/learn attitude: "Oh, wow! My favorite!" (joy) "I am feeling quite full." (neutral assessment of situation) "But I think I have room for a bite or two. I'll have a slice of cake." (pleasure and anticipation of the taste) The first bite of cake is eaten slowly, and the diner savors every morsel. When you slowly savor a food, often you will find that one or two bites are satisfying. Let's say, though, that this naturally slim person got distracted and didn't stop eating after the two bites she planned to eat. "I can't believe I ate that whole piece of cake! I must not have been paying attention." (lesson) "I don't like feeling this stuffed at all!" (acknowledgment of feelings, without judgment) "Next time I'm going to pay more attention." (lesson) or "Next time I'm going to order dessert before my meal." (lesson) or "Next time I'm going to check the dessert cart and not order such a big meal if they have my favorite dessert." (lesson) All three are loving, caring choices. The cake was thoroughly enjoyed by the diner up until the time she ceased to pay attention; then her lack of attention brought her a bit of pain or discomfort. Was that bad? No! Discomfort is the stimulus that causes us to move and grow.

On your journey to becoming naturally slim, allow yourself to make mistakes without judgment or guilt. Proceed diligently on your journey without a worry about when it will end. Even if you make the same mistakes over and over, stand back, look at what you're doing with curiosity, and see what is there for you to learn. When you truly learn the lesson in your heart, not just in your head, you will no longer need to repeat that mistake.

I read the following wisdom in a greeting card years ago: "Yesterday is history; tomorrow is mystery; today is a gift; that is why they call it the present."

> When you are eating—Be Here Now! without judgment.
>
> When you are reading—Be Here Now! without judgment.
>
> When you are feeling fat and miserable—Be Here Now! without judgment.
>
> When you are feeling loved and special—Be Here Now! without judgment.

Only through attention to our actions and feelings can we know ourselves and begin to grow and change.

Opportunities for Growth

Awareness

- Make a decision to focus your attention one day a week on all of the thought energy you spend judging yourself, feeling guilty, and worrying. See if just becoming aware might allow you to change those thoughts.

- Put a sign at your desk and in your car and in your kitchen: "Guilt and worry are a waste of my time and energy" or (my favorite sign, short and sweet) "BE HERE NOW!"

- Make a list of foods you feel are "good" or "bad" and begin to attach neutral feelings to them. For example, you can replace "ice cream is bad" with "ice cream is cold." Before you are able to choose food for health, you will need to drop your judgments of them as good or bad.

- Go grocery shopping and buy foods without judgment— there are no good or bad foods. Begin to bring food into the house that you previously have judged "bad" and release that judgment. Bring in healthy foods you have judged as boring and release that judgment. If bringing in certain foods sends you into gut-wrenching fear, then don't buy them. However, realize there is something to learn from that fear. Food of any kind need not be a source of fear. Find out what is fearsome for you about that food and begin to release those fears.

Introspection

- Keep a small spiral notebook in your pocket or purse. Before, during, or after eating, note what you were eating and how you felt when you were done. No judgment! If you felt empty and unsatisfied after a healthy serving of tofu fritter, write it down. If you felt warm and fuzzy and almost had an orgasm after a hot fudge banana split, write it down. If you weren't hungry at all and binged on the leftover cold pizza in the refrigerator because you were lonesome and now you feel like a fat toad, write it down. You will never learn what is contributing to your inability to be as slim as you were meant to be unless you stop judging what you're doing, stop burying your feelings, and shine a light on your relationship with food.

Old Beliefs to Let Go

- I need to be right.

- It is good to feel guilty.

- Worrying is a necessary part of life.

- I eat a lot of bad foods.

New Beliefs to Embrace

- I accept myself without judgment.

- I forgive myself any wrongs that have caused me hurt.

- I release myself from the need to feel guilty.

- I chose foods to eat that enhance my health.

Vividly Imagine

- Imagine a world without judgment, guilt, or worry. Imagine your own mind without judgment, guilt, or worry. What would you think about all day?

Patterns for Action

- Pick one specific judgment you have about a person, place, or thing that you would like to be nonjudgmental about. Be committed to catching yourself in judgment and guilt. Plan what to do instead.

Additional Reading

Dyer, Wayne, Ph.D. *Your Erroneous Zones*. New York: Harper and Row, 1976.

Roger, John, and Peter McWilliams. *You Can't Afford the Luxury of a Negative Thought*. Los Angeles: Prelude Press, 1988.

SEVEN

Habit 4: Trust Your Body

You are not meant to live in fear of your own body. Know that your body, mind, and spirit are always working on your behalf. Even if you are deeply involved in emotional eating, it is not because your body is betraying you; it is because right now you know no other way to comfort yourself.

ONE OF THE MOST remarkable things we noticed in our interviews with naturally slim people was the ease with which they discussed their bodies and their eating habits. There was no embarrassment, no secrets, no lies or smoke screens. There was an air of comfort, ease, and confidence in their relationship with their physical bodies. Naturally slim people *trust* their bodies. Chronic dieters and unnaturally slim people don't.

Each and every one of us was born with a marvelously adaptable body. We don't even have to think about 90 percent of the functions that are going on at any given time. Our hearts beat, our lungs breathe, our liver and kidneys filter and detoxify our blood, our eyes see, our ears hear, and on and on without any conscious thought on our part. We all have a hunger center and a satiety center located in the hypothalamic portion of our brain.

We have a very sophisticated network of sensors that notifies our hunger center when blood levels of glucose, amino acids (the building blocks of protein), or fats drop below an acceptable level. Our bodies know when they are hungry, and they tell us so. Our bodies know when they are satisfied, and they tell us so. Our bodies know what kind of fuel they need, and tell us what that is. All we have to do is listen, trust, and follow through.

Imagine what it would be like to wake up each morning not quite sure if your heart would keep beating or your eyes would keep seeing. You would spend most of your day in fear and indecision, not sure if you should drive the car, go to work, or stay home and concentrate on your unreliable organs, hoping that if you paid close attention to them you could keep them working. It would be a life filled with constant fear and time for little else. Many people who are overweight or have lost weight dieting walk around with that depth of fear, wondering if they are eating the right thing, afraid that they will break out in fat at any moment; weighing themselves one, two, or even three times a day. They are obsessed with thoughts about their body and its size, leaving time for little else. They live in a constant state of fear because they feel they cannot trust their bodies.

An important part of becoming naturally slim is developing trust in your own body. Doing this will require an investment of time and attention. However, it will be one of the best investments you have ever made. When you are able to trust your body, you can wake up in the morning and decide if you are hungry, if you want a large or a small breakfast, if you want to eat only half of what you prepared, or if you are still hungry and need a second serving. No food plans, no menus—it all sounds so . . . so . . . *natural*, doesn't it? Trusting your own body means depending on it, relying on it, having a firm belief in its powers and its truthfulness. Very few people who have wrestled with being overweight can honestly say they feel this way about their bodies.

We Are Born Trusting Our Bodies; Fear Is Learned

Trust in a relationship—any relationship, even our relationship with our own bodies—is a very delicate thing. From an early age we have been taught, by well-meaning adults, to fear and distrust many persons, places, and things. As innocent, trusting, loving children we grow up surrounded by fears and warnings. Trust becomes an unaffordable luxury. If we trust, we may get hurt or killed, brokenhearted, or fat. The innate trust we had in our bodies as children becomes suspect, especially under parental prodding about food and weight: "Clean your plate." "I don't care if you're not hungry; eat your vegetables." "Don't eat that cookie; you'll spoil your dinner." "Stay away from that candy; it will make you fat." "You're getting a little chubby; maybe you better skip dessert." These admonitions start to erode children's body trust.

In addition we hear our sisters or mothers talk endlessly about how "fat" they are and the latest diet they are on. Television, movies, and magazines are filled with pictures of women with bodies we have not seen in the real world. Young girls quickly surmise that because it is on TV it must be the ideal body and decide they want theirs to look that way too. Never mind that the female body type that we see in the media 99 percent of our waking hours is a body type that only 1 percent of the population can maintain naturally. This leads to all kinds of unnatural efforts by teens and adults to achieve a body size that is totally unrealistic when their genetic makeup, body type, and metabolism are taken into consideration. Their efforts may include anorexia, bulimia, chronic dieting, and exercise addiction.

We trust the media, our doctors, and our parents, so we diet until we achieve some arbitrary standard. Then, slowly but surely, we gain all the weight back. Ironically, instead of distrusting the people who sent us looking for that ideal body, we turn our distrust on ourselves! Why do we trust those that send us on wild goose chases and distrust ourselves? The answer is clear: low self-worth and inadequate love and respect for ourselves as intelligent, instinctual human beings. We have very strong underlying beliefs that we are weak and that we can't possibly know enough to determine the best way to reduce our body fat, so we turn to someone else—we turn to *everyone* else besides the people who know us best, ourselves.

Please understand that I am not saying advice from other people is totally useless. If I believed that, I wouldn't be writing this book. Advice, however, that ignores you as a person possessing intelligence, instincts, and freedom of choice is misdirected advice. Trust the person who wants to support your personal growth, not the person who wants you to do what he or she tells you without using your intuition and self-knowledge.

Take Your Eyes and Your Mind Off the Scale!

Naturally slim people trust their bodies. They eat when hungry, they eat what they like, they stop eating when satisfied, and they weigh themselves infrequently. They do not believe that they will immediately put on fat if they eat a piece of cheesecake. They do not believe that if the scale goes up two pounds they are on their way to obesity. When they do weigh themselves, they pay attention to the number only as it fits into a long-term pattern. When they look at the scale, they think, I feel fine, my clothes fit well, and I don't think an increase of two pounds means anything, or, I expect my weight to fluctuate two to five pounds, and if it fluctuates more than that I'll start to pay closer attention to what I'm eating.

We strongly encourage you to stop weighing yourself so frequently. Every three to six months is more than enough. In fact if you have access to a nutritionist or a local chapter of the American Heart Association, you're better off having someone who is trained to do so measure your body fat percentage. Percent body fat is a more accurate reflection of the process of becoming naturally slim than measuring pounds. During this process you are burning excess body fat, not losing weight. Actually, the fit of your clothes will also tell the story. I was totally amazed when I went from fall to spring without losing a pound but found that all my spring clothes were loose. This is the kind of weight loss that occurs when you are becoming naturally slim. It is slow, consistent, and all fat. You don't want just weight loss, which can include water loss and muscle loss as well. Whether it is pounds or percent body fat, however, the important thing is to detach yourself from a number and make choices toward health in each present moment.

Your Body Is Normal and Programmed to Preserve Your Life

We all depend on our bodies to function reliably and get our minds and spirits through the day. That reliance means we need to trust the body to do its job well. Trust can make us feel vulnerable, especially when we must trust something outside ourselves, but I'm asking you to trust *yourself*. "How can I trust my body?" you might ask. "Look at the size of it. I eat so very little and yet I stay so very big. There must be something wrong with me." Please understand that being overweight and needing very few calories to stay that way does not mean your body has betrayed you. Your body has done very reliably what it is designed to do. It has taken calories you have eaten in excess of the calories you have burned and stored them as fat. It has also stored fat and reduced your metabolic rate in response to being starved.

Dieting is starvation to your body. Your body is being given so little food to sustain its functions that it must digest some of itself—important lean body mass like muscle tissue as well as fat. What the body chooses to burn for fuel when it is starving depends on what type of fuel it is being fed and how restricted the total intake is. The more severely restricted the diet, the more muscle loss there will be. The more muscle loss there is, the less ability you have to burn calories and the easier it is to become fat.

The more frequently and severely you have dieted, the greater your weight gain and the more time it will take to return to your predieting leanness and metabolism. That is not your body's fault; it is just a physiological fact. So please trust your body, and understand that the slower the weight loss, the greater the guarantee that it will be permanent.

I can hear some of you saying right now, "OK, OK, maybe my body does know what it's doing somewhere under all this fat, but what about the way I eat sometimes? I know I can't trust myself around a box of chocolates or a bowl of chips . . . and that's a fact! When I'm around certain foods, I'm like an addict— I can't stop!" Another facet of trust is knowing that your body is not by nature addicted to foods. Your reactions to and cravings for certain foods have either a physiological or a psychological basis. You can learn from them and grow and change because of them. If you just decide arbitrarily that you are weak-willed and addicted to potato chips and that you will never have them in the house, you are deciding on a solution before you really understand the problem. When you are away from home and someone has potato chips in the house, what will happen? If you do decide to buy just one bag and take it home, what will happen? You will probably overeat the chips because (1) you have deprived yourself of them and (2) you never addressed the possible reasons for your craving.

Food Cravings Are Messages, Not Moral Weaknesses

When dealing with compulsive eating of various foods, you can try several approaches: First, get rid of the belief "When I am around potato chips, I have no control; I can't stop eating them." Replace that belief with "Potato chips are just another food. They mean nothing to me. When I am around potato chips, I can take them or leave them." If you continue to say that you are addicted to potato chips, you will be, because your mind knows no other program. It is operating on the program that says you are addicted, and addiction means anytime you see chips you eat them. This program totally bypasses your normal regulatory impulses of hunger and satiety. You can begin to change this belief by repeating the new positive statement to yourself in the mirror several times a day, or more efficiently you can change the belief by doing the Psych-K balance taught in Chapter 17.

Second, evaluate your nutritional intake. Potato chips are salty, crunchy, oily carbohydrates. Has your diet been deficient in any of these nutrients, tastes, or textures? If the salt is the appealing part, what has your water intake been? The body uses salt to hold on to water when it is not getting enough. So if you have ignored your body's need for $1^{1}/_{2}$ liters of water per day, it may now be craving salt to hold on to the water it has. Is it summer? Do you sweat a lot? Have you been out in the sun or exercising or even doing a lot of thinking? Water is crucial. Do you drink mostly caffeinated beverages like cola, black tea, and coffee? These beverages actually cause diuresis, which means the caffeine increases water loss through your kidneys so that you lose each ounce you take in. Have you been outdoors and gotten sunshine on a regular basis? One study has linked carbohydrate craving to lack of exposure to full-spectrum light.

Third, ask yourself, "If I am a pleasure-seeking being, what pleasures am I obtaining from this habit? Maybe I like hearing the crunch. Maybe it reminds me of the ones my dad used to bring me or all the fun parties I went to in high school. Or maybe I just like that feeling of a full tummy or doing something I know I shouldn't be doing. Or maybe I do it to defy those thin people."

Fourth, rationally look at the pleasures and start giving yourself those pleasures—fun, love, security, joy, danger, assertiveness—in other ways so that you don't have to use potato chips to get them. Then begin to look at the downside of eating the potato chips when you aren't hungry and see if the painful aspects outweigh the pleasures. But remember, eating potato chips when you are not hungry is filling some sort of physiological or psychological need. You must determine what those needs are and meet them in some other way before you let go of the chips. If you do not, you may end up substituting some other habit that is just as unhealthy, like the person who gives up cigarettes and takes up food as a substitute. This happens frequently when a habit is broken without addressing the needs that the habit was filling.

Food Sensitivities

Much research has shown that often people become "addicted" to foods they are sensitive to. They will develop cravings for milk, cheese, wheat, or eggs and actually experience a type of withdrawal when the foods are removed from their diet. When the foods are removed for a sufficient period of time, around 90 days, they often can be reintroduced in limited amounts as long as they are not consumed every day. For more information about food sensitivities, consult a nutritionist who is experienced in that area and read the book by Dr. Braly listed at the end of this chapter.

I hope you can see that your body, mind, and spirit are always looking out for your best interest. If you need love and the only way you know right now to get it is by eating chocolate, then your mind will send you to eat chocolate. Your body would rather not do this from a physiological standpoint because chocolate has very limited nutritional value. However, the need for love, comfort, and safety can override your body's innate nutritional wisdom. If you begin to meet your need for love, comfort, and safety in other ways, your mind will allow your body's natural wisdom about food to shine through. That might mean having chocolate once in a while but not to excess. No one is born with an innate need for chocolate; that is a learned desire. Neither, however, is chocolate bad in and of itself. It's just that eating it when you're not hungry or eating it for emotional reasons will contribute to excess body fat.

Trust that anything you do that appears on the surface to be working against your own health is answering a real psychological or physiological need and thus serving your highest interest. Be an ever zealous detective to identify and fill those needs. If you nurture your mind and spirit directly, you won't have to do so with food. When you stop using food to fill psychological needs, you can begin to use it to feed your body, which is the way it is supposed to be. Trust that if you stay in the process of becoming healthy in body, mind, and spirit, you will rediscover all the instincts your body has to help you reach your optimal body weight and stay there for life.

One of the ways that trust in your body can be reinforced is to give yourself as many opportunities to experience trust as possible. When we talk about hunger and satisfaction in the next few chapters, it is crucial to allow yourself to get hungry and then feed yourself in a gentle, healthy manner. Just like an infant who develops trust in the world by crying for food and getting fed, every time you allow yourself the gentle trusting experience of eating when you are hungry and eating what you want, you reinforce a trusting relationship with your body's natural hunger signals.

Opportunities for Growth

Awareness

- Look up the word *trust* in a dictionary and thesaurus to get a true feeling for what it means to you.

- Write down or make a mental list of all of the things you trust your body to do for you every day. Isn't it possible that it also can be trusted to let you know when and what to eat?

- What foods do you find yourself craving and when? Write them down (No judgment, detective!). See if you can figure out what needs they are meeting, either physiologically or psychologically.

- How many times a day or week do you weigh yourself? Why? How would your day change if you decided not to weigh yourself?

Introspection

- How many ways do you have for taking care of yourself, making yourself feel safe and loved, besides food?

- Are you willing to begin building some new ways to care for yourself? Do you make excuses like having no time, no energy, or not knowing how?

Old Beliefs to Let Go

- My body can't be trusted.

- If I look at a dessert, I will gain weight.

- I must weigh myself every day, or my weight will get out of control.

- I can't have _____ (chips, cookies, candy, other) in the house or I will eat them all.

New Beliefs to Embrace

- I am normal.

- I trust my body and all of my natural instincts to move me toward health.

- I trust myself to choose healthy, nutritious food to eat.

- My weight is an insignificant number.

Vividly Imagine

- Imagine yourself totally trusting your natural instincts. What would you buy at the store? What would your kitchen cabinets look like? Visualize yourself standing in front of your most feared food, with no reaction, no fear.

Patterns for Action

- Begin to release your attachments to your bathroom scale,

with the goal of eventually getting rid of it. Put a piece of tape over the readout with a weight that you enjoy printed on it, then when you weigh yourself you will always be pleased. Consider the possibility of weighing yourself in Denver versus Miami. Would you weigh less in the mile-high city? Or what about the moon? Wouldn't your weight be considerably less there? Heaven forbid that you might lose an arm in an accident, but you certainly would weigh less, right? Next time you are at the doctor's office, ask why they need your weight. If it is not to determine a medication dosage, it is probably unnecessary. Or get weighed facing away from the scale so you don't have to see the number, or wear your coat, hat, and purse and really confuse them.

- The next time you find yourself eating something "for no good reason," there probably is a good reason. Without judgment, stop and write down the answers to these questions: What am I getting out of eating this? Physically? Emotionally? Have I been missing something in my regular meals? Have I been neglecting to feed myself emotionally? Is there any other way I can get what I need without using food? Even if you choose to continue eating that food, at least you are doing it with awareness. You will begin to see patterns in your eating behaviors that will give you concrete areas to work on.

Additional Reading

Braly, James, M.D. *Dr. Braly's Food Allergy and Nutrition Revolution.* New Canaan, Keats, 1992.

Hirschmann, Jane, and Carol Munter. *When Women Stop Hating Their Bodies.* New York: Fawcett Columbine, 1995.

Jeffers, Susan, Ph.D. *Feel the Fear and Do It Anyway.* New York: Fawcett Columbine, 1987.

EIGHT

Habit 5: Eat When You're Hungry

*To feel pleasantly hungry and to satisfy
that hunger is a gesture of self-love we can
repeat over and over. Hunger is not the
villain; it is ignorance and fear of our
hunger that lead us astray.*

WHEN CHRONIC DIETERS are asked the question "When do you eat?" the responses go something like this: "I eat at mealtime." "I eat when I'm depressed." "I eat when I'm tired." "I eat when I'm bored." "I eat before I go to bed." "I eat when I'm angry." "I eat when I don't feel good." When we asked the same question of naturally slim people, their answer was unanimous: "I eat when I'm hungry." What a simple but wondrous enlightenment this is for all of us. What would it be like just to eat when you're hungry? What would it be like just to stop eating when you are satisfied? That sounds too simple, you might say.

It *is* simple, yet it is the cornerstone of becoming naturally slim. Remember that naturally instinctive infant we talked about in Chapter 2? He knew when he was hungry, and he made darn sure he got something to eat. We all have the natural instinct to feed ourselves when we are hungry. If we didn't, we would die of starvation. However, the time since we were intimately in tune with our physical hunger and could differentiate it from psychological hunger can be counted in decades for some of us!

It is quite common for weight loss programs to advertise, "On our program you will never be hungry!" as if hunger were some sort of sinister villain to be avoided at all costs. If you are never hungry, how will you know when to eat? When the program director tells you that you can? When a book or magazine article tells you that you should? Do you really think that it is your fate to spend your life having someone else tell you when, where, what, and how much to eat?

If so, go back to Chapter 5 and work on your self-esteem until you begin to feel that you have the right and the intelligence to learn about your own body and select healthy foods for it. Ask yourself how much of the rest of your life you will live according to what other people tell you to do. If you are looking for a book that will tell you exactly what to eat on which day, you're in the wrong place. This book is about self-love, self-responsibility, freedom, and choices.

If you aren't going to rely on a diet program to tell you when to eat, who *do* you rely on? The answer, of course, is yourself. Your hunger signals, as personal as they are to each and every one of you, will work for you just as they work for the naturally slim person. But if they are to work for you, you must first be able to recognize them. You must become acquainted with them, view them as a friend, and become intimately aware of what they are telling you. When was the last time you felt hungry? When was the last time you felt hungry without feeling ravenous? Did you know that there are degrees of hunger and there are types of hunger? Did you know that it is entirely possible to be hungry one hour after a big meal if the meal was not balanced, if it contained a lot of sugar, alcohol, or white flour, or if it did not meet your body's nutritional needs?

Some overweight people think they are going crazy or that they must have some psychological problem because they are driven to the refrigerator two hours after a good-sized meal. No, they are not crazy; their bodies are just telling them, "Yes, you fed your stomach, and it is full, but what I really need right now has nothing to do with what you ate." Maybe you ate a huge salad and your body is hungry for some protein. Maybe you had bacon and eggs and toast and your body is hungry for vitamin C, vitamin A, and beta-carotene. Maybe you had pasta and dessert, and you oversecreted insulin in response to these simple carbohydrates (75 percent of the population does). Now you feel hungry, maybe even faint, because your blood sugar is so low. These are all normal physiologic occurrences. Once you begin to recognize your hunger signals and relate them to needing fuel for your body, you can begin to discern what kind of fuel you should put in. When you begin balancing your diet with high-quality nutritious food, your hunger will be more balanced also. In this chapter we will talk about hunger. In Chapter 12 we will discuss how to choose what kinds of food to put into your fuel tank.

In our experience three different types of hunger actually operate in most people: (1) physical hunger, (2) nutrient hunger, and (3) psychological hunger. In naturally slim people, the first two are intimately linked. However, in those of us who have been out of tune with our hunger signals for years and even decades it is important to understand all three.

Physical Hunger

Physical hunger is a strong desire for food that is usually associated with a number of objective sensations. The sensations may be as subtle as a decrease in ability to focus and concentrate, a lack of energy or drive, or a feeling of tenseness or restlessness. Some people describe a strange feeling throughout their entire body or a twitteriness. These subtle feelings will often be followed by the more noticeable feelings of hunger contractions, a tight kind of gnawing feeling or growling in the stomach. Hunger contractions are the strongest in young healthy people, and their intensity is greatly increased by a low level of blood sugar. All of these feelings are associated with the body's need for regular nourishment. Low blood sugar, as well as decreased levels of other nutrients, stimulates the feeding center in the hypothalamus, which is located in the upper portion of the brain stem. What is important to remember is that even people without stomachs experience physical hunger. We all do; it is our inborn drive to seek food and maintain life.

Still, we are going to focus on the stomach when we talk about physical hunger because the sensations felt in the stomach are fairly strong and somewhat familiar to people. When you are ready, take hunger a step further and notice what other bodily sensations accompany it. Do you get irritable and lose focus on what you're doing before you get that growl in your stomach? Do you feel very little in your stomach until you are almost faint? Your hunger sensations are personal. Get to know them.

The first step in the process of becoming tuned in to your physical hunger signals is to allow yourself to get hungry. Promise yourself you will eat something after you get hungry, that you will not let yourself become ravenous, but that in the interest of becoming naturally slim or what we call a *natural instinctive eater* you need to stop eating just "because it is time to eat." You need to begin eating when you are hungry. Part of developing a trusting relationship with your body is letting your body know that you are paying attention on a regular basis, that you will recognize its hunger signals.

Just like any other skill, getting good at recognizing your hunger signals takes practice. Keep a little spiral notebook in your pocket and make some notes. Pretend you are a scientist on a fascinating trek to rediscover your natural instincts. Instead of seeing note-keeping as drudgery, approach it with an attitude of curiosity and wonder, like an infant who has just discovered her toes. Becoming aware of your own body is a kind and loving thing to do for yourself. If you are saying, "I don't have time," go back to Habit 1 and Habit 2. If health is a priority in your life and you love yourself, you will find the time. We're talking about less than 30 seconds four to eight times a day. What a small investment to make in your health!

Hunger Awareness Training

Here is a typical morning routine for someone in hunger aware-ness training: Wake up in the morning, go to the rest room, and have one or two small glasses of water (you've just gone six to eight hours without any water, and you don't want to confuse thirst and hunger). Proceed with brushing your teeth and so on and then, before you go to the kitchen, before you grab your coffee or what-ever your routine is, *stop*. Start to break your unconscious habits by breaking your routine. Close your eyes, take a deep breath, and focus on your stomach. Ask yourself, "Am I hungry?" It is some-times useful to use a hunger rating scale when you start out. One that our clients find very helpful is presented in Figure 2.

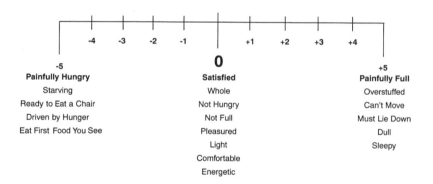

Figure 2. Hunger–Satisfaction Scale

As you can see in Figure 2, zero equals satisfied, no feeling, not empty, not full, just there. Moving toward the plus side are degrees of fullness. Moving toward the minus side are degrees of physical hunger. Focus on your stomach and note where you are on the scale. If you're on the plus side (maybe you ate dinner at 10:00 last night?), your stomach is not signaling hunger. If you're at zero, check again later. If you are at −4 or −5, head for the kitchen immediately. If you're at −1 or −2, you can wait a little while to eat, but don't wait too long. If you wait to eat until you are at −4 or −5, it will be harder to control the amounts you eat and you will not be supporting a trusting relationship with your body. It will continue to wonder, "Is she always going to wait to feed me until I'm ravenous?"

Forget about all that hype that breakfast is the most important meal of the day. If you are not hungry, don't eat. However, anticipate that you may indeed be hungry in an hour or two and plan how you can meet your body's need for food at that time. Pack yourself something to eat that is nutritious and balanced, with carbohydrates, protein, and a small amount of fat, not a few carrot sticks or a bag of potato chips just to stop the growling. A sandwich on whole-grain bread or some fruit complemented with a handful of nuts or seeds can fill the bill nicely. Remember, there are no rules about where and when you can eat. If you are really hungry at 10:00 A.M. in the middle of your workday, take out your sandwich and eat it. Until you recognize and honor your body's hunger signals, you will be constantly at war with yourself. Tell the boss you have a medical condition or go outside or to the rest room—do whatever you have to do.

If you tune in to your body at your usual mealtime and you are not hungry but you choose to eat anyway, remember: no judgment, no guilt, and no self-flagellation. You are not "doing it wrong," and no, you have not blown another weight loss program. When you are ready, you will decide to do it differently, one meal, one day at a time.

See yourself as a scientist would. Be aware of your behavior, maintain your curiosity, and wonder, "Why did I do that?" Make a note of it in your little spiral notebook and see how many times a day or week you do that. Use it as a learning experience. Some of our clients who use computers in their job keep a file for these kinds of notes.

When you start out, you may find yourself eating often when you are not physically hungry. That's to be expected—it's one of the reasons you have had difficulty maintaining your naturally slim body. But at least now you are *aware* of it. Awareness is the very first step toward change and growth. You cannot make healthful changes if you are not even aware of what you are doing now that is unhealthy. Most naturally slim people eat some sort of breakfast, sometimes large, sometimes small. They eat the breakfast because they are hungry, not because it is breakfast time. If you are not hungry at all in the morning or feel on the plus side, start to look at the amount of eating you do in the evening. I went for years never eating breakfast or lunch but eating continuously from 4:00 P.M. until midnight. Of course I wasn't hungry in the morning!

Don't Be Afraid to Be Hungry

Allow yourself to feel physical hunger. Don't be afraid of it. Notice the first twinge of hunger, then let it go for a while. How do you feel? Get to know what happens if you let your hunger go too long. If you feed yourself small amounts of nutritious food when you are hungry, you may feel hunger every three hours or so. If you take just a bite or two of something, you may be hungry every hour. If you eat a very filling lunch, you may not be hungry for five hours. This is why no one can really tell you exactly how much and when to eat. Only your body knows what it needs.

There are times during your hunger awareness training that you may become frustrated because you get very hungry at 3:00 P.M., and you eat, but you were supposed to go out to dinner at 5:00 P.M. and you are not the least bit hungry! In time you will learn to snack on something small if you have plans for dinner. However, it is a great learning experience to go out to dinner when you are not hungry. What do you do? Do you eat anyway, in violation of your own body signals? Do you have just water? Do you order dinner, pick at it, and then take it home? The goal is to be comfortable enough with yourself, your health, and the choice not to eat if you're not hungry. A naturally slim person would never think of eating dinner just because he paid for it or because people would look at him funny if he didn't.

Nutrient Hunger

If you find yourself in the kitchen and check in with your stomach, you may discover you're not really hungry but still have a strong desire to eat something. You may be experiencing either nutrient hunger or psychological hunger, and it is important to begin to differentiate between the two. When you experience nutrient hunger, often your stomach isn't empty. It has had enough food bulkwise, but your body is saying it needs something very specific, something it hasn't had enough of in the last day or so. You may get a craving for a very specific food or just a general feeling that something is missing, that you need something very specific to "hit the spot." Standing in the kitchen, combing through the cabinets and refrigerator looking for that specific food, is actually a modern version of an ancient activity called *foraging*. The difference is that foraging through our kitchens is often like foraging through a vast wasteland. The preponderance of dead, processed, preserved, and nutritionally empty products we stock gives us little chance to accurately assess our nutrient hunger and satisfy it with the nutrients we need. We look and look, and nothing appeals to us, so we just grab whatever is there, leaving us fed but not nourished. This is why it is important to take some time to (1) understand basic nutrition and know what types of nutrients your body needs so that you know what it may not have had; (2) tune in to what you're hungry for *before* you go into a kitchen full of limited choices; and (3) keep a wide variety of nutritious foods available. Only then will you be able to match what you eat with what your body wants.

If you made a strange sigh or a sound rather like "ugh" when I mentioned nutrition, think of it this way: Would you put leaded gas in a car that requires unleaded gas? Heavens no! The car would run poorly, and parts of it would be damaged. You know what kind of fuel your car needs to run. Isn't it worth a bit of your time to understand what your body needs to run well?

Understanding basic nutrition does not mean that you have to become obsessed with it. You can be informed and well nourished and slim without being a "health nut." Becoming obsessed with nutrition may be healthier than being obsessed with dieting, but it is equally unsound when it comes to living a balanced life.

Once you understand what a balanced nutritious diet is, you

can begin to match up your mysterious hungers with various nutrients that are missing from your diet. For example, say you had a bowl of cereal and milk, an orange, and a cup of coffee for breakfast, and you even took your vitamins. One or two hours later you begin to feel uncomfortable, irritable. Your stomach isn't growling, but you feel you need something to eat. Before you head for the doughnut box, think about what you had for breakfast. This particular breakfast was very low in protein and high in carbohydrate. This, together with the caffeine in the coffee, which can lower your blood sugar, indicates that a high-protein snack with a little carbohydrate would be the best thing to eat. That means something besides a doughnut. Where do you get protein on a coffee break? It's not so easy. Here is where planning ahead and keeping a hard-boiled egg, cheese and crackers, peanut butter, or something similar available will be very helpful. Also, begin to balance your breakfast by adding protein: eggs, meat, cheese (Chapter 18 will cover nutrition in detail).

One tip about mornings: Filling your stomach with a cup or two of coffee can temporarily blunt hunger signals that will reappear with a vengeance later. Also, caffeine may wake you up, but it can also cause your blood sugar to drop dramatically, leaving you feeling hungry and weak, especially if you haven't eaten anything. Finally, caffeine also acts as a mild diuretic, which will leave your body needing increased water intake. Keeping yourself well hydrated is one of the best ways to nourish your body. Are we telling you not to drink coffee? Are we telling you to drink only decaf? No, we are giving you information about how coffee and specifically caffeine can interfere with your natural physical signals. You may decide in the future that you want to reduce that interference. It is always your choice. If it were not your choice, you would resent the change and see it as a restriction to your freedom. I used to start my day with two cups of coffee with sugar and creamer and nothing else, and by 10:30 I would feel weak and shaky. I decided to let go of caffeine rather than coffee. The first time I switched to decaf I had severe headaches and felt as if I couldn't get moving in the morning, so I quit. The next time, I just started mixing decaf and regular coffee, gradually increasing the amount of decaf over several weeks. By the end of the month I was on all decaf, and I didn't even know the difference—except, of course, my midmorning faintness was gone.

Making changes gradually and pleasurably is important. Take cozy habits you enjoy such as your morning coffee and gradually turn them into something a bit healthier for yourself. The more you treat yourself lovingly during the change process, the more motivated you will be to continue. Over a year's time my coffee habit went from caffeinated to decaffeinated to a chai (an Indian tea with milk, honey, and spices) and protein powder shake. It was a gradual change, and I did it for my health but also because I enjoyed it. I did not do it because some book said I should. My morning habit also includes sitting with my warm cup on the sofa, reading or looking out the window while everyone in the house is still asleep. I have not changed that part of the habit one bit. My enjoyment is in the moment, not just in what I am drinking.

If you find yourself looking for something to eat and you are not really physically hungry, check yourself for nutrient hunger. What did you eat last? Was it balanced? Have you had anything fresh to eat today? Any fruits or vegetables? These are the most common sources of nutrients left out of our daily food intake. In this day and age of microwaves and fast food, you may find you have gone for days without having fresh foods, which are the mainstay of a healthy diet. Also check your emotional state. If you are not hungry, but you recently experienced some sort of emotional upset, anxiety, sadness, or frustration, you may be psychologically hungry. If you are drawn to nutrient-challenged foods like sweets, creamy things, or chips, it's a pretty good bet that you are not experiencing nutrient hunger. True nutrient hunger may tell you a nice crispy salad is exactly what you want. This rarely happens with psychological hunger.

Psychological Hunger

Quite simply, psychological hunger is in your head and in your heart. It is a drive to eat food for reasons that have absolutely nothing to do with the physical nourishment of your body. Love, comfort, and food have been closely linked from the time we were first held and fed from breast or bottle. The warmth, the sweetness, the creaminess of our infant feedings are intimately connected with comfort and soothing in our minds. Didn't being fed soothe those terrible hunger pains? Didn't being fed mean being held and feeling safe and secure and totally fulfilled? As infants we were easily pleased; happiness truly was a full belly.

These connections are not easily forgotten, and there will always be foods in our life that we associate with comfort. There will always be meals that are so much more than physically satisfying because they were made with love. Does Mom's apple pie truly taste better than the bakery's because of the ingredients or because of the love that is baked into it? In our quest for good nutrition and our understanding that food is the fuel that runs our physical body, we do not want to eliminate the psychological satisfaction that certain foods at certain times and in certain kitchens may bring to us. What we do want to do is to put that into perspective.

If you have a habit of feeding your psychological hungers with physical food, you place yourself in double jeopardy. Not only do you inadequately meet your psychological needs but you become fat in the process! So, as we talked about in Chapter 1, you get sucked into a negative spiral of feeling unhappy and eating more, becoming fatter, and feeling even worse. For these reasons it is important to begin identifying your psychological and emotional hungers and to feed them with nonfood nurturing. This, like any other learning process, cannot be done in one fell swoop. It is a process, a series of steps. Deciding that every time you find yourself eating ice cream because you are lonely you will stop and call a friend instead is laudable but not very realistic.

The very first step is to recognize that you have feelings to begin with. Whether you eat ice cream or call a friend, your action is an attempt to feel loneliness as little as possible and for the shortest time. You perceive this feeling as painful and want to make the pain stop. When you stuff yourself with food over a psychological dilemma, you trade the loneliness—or sadness, anger, and so on—for temporary pleasure (the first two bites) and then guilt over overeating. Overweight people don't mind feeling guilty—they're used to that. Guilt is a comfortable, familiar feeling, one that they think they deserve, because very few of them love themselves enough to know that they deserve better.

What might happen if you honored your feelings? What might happen if you considered being sad OK; if you said to yourself, "I won't die if I feel sad, and maybe I can learn something about myself if I respect my sadness"? I'm not suggesting that you should spend weeks wallowing in sadness. If you are stuck feeling that sad for that long, it might be advisable to seek professional help. I will tell you, though, that some of my most profound insights have come to me after I allowed myself to cry good and hard. I have also noticed that not once did I receive a startling insight after consuming a half gallon of ice cream. Consider honoring your feelings; consider them messengers bearing the news that there is a conflict between your spirit self and the way you are leading some part of your life. Your emotions are a tap on the shoulder. Don't ignore them; don't just stuff them down with food. Bring them out in the open, feel them deeply, and then ask yourself for insight so that you can move on. When you begin recognizing your psychological and emotional needs and taking care of them, you will no longer need to feed them with food.

You have the time to do this, one day, one episode, one feeling at a time. Taking the time to sit with your feelings is kind, loving, and healthy and an important part of becoming naturally slim. Slim people have just as many feelings as you do. They just handle them in ways that don't involve food. Begin to recognize when you are emotionally or spiritually hungry. Realize that you are in need of something that has nothing to do with food and that no matter how much you eat, it will never fill that need.

As you recognize your nonphysical hungers, you may be tempted to berate yourself or feel that you are weak-willed because you continue to meet your emotional needs with food. Don't berate yourself; realize that up until now you have been comforting yourself the only way you knew how. Say this to yourself, but also decide that you will begin to learn other ways to comfort yourself and that you will begin to fill up your emotional or spiritual tank on a regular basis so that you aren't so emotionally starved that you make unhealthy choices.

What Do Naturally Slim People Do When They Need Comfort?

We asked naturally slim people whether they ever used food to comfort themselves, and if not what they did instead. Approximately 50 percent said they rarely or never used food to comfort themselves. The other 50 percent said they sometimes used food to comfort themselves. None of the naturally slim people we talked to answered that they used food regularly, often, or always for comfort. Here are some of their answers:

JT: "I rarely, really never, use food to comfort myself. When I need comfort, I read or write."

LW: "Sometimes I'll have hot tea, milk and cookies, or a cappuccino for comfort. Usually I do something like take a bubble bath, read, get a manicure or pedicure, or just curl up in bed and watch TV."

NA: "I rarely turn to food for comfort. Hot tea, a hot bath, or a movie would be my choice for comfort."

GG: "I never eat for comfort, but I will have a drink once in a while."

ST: "I rarely eat for comfort. I prefer to read, listen to music, or meditate. On the rare occasions I do use food, I usually choose chips or chocolate, but not large amounts."

MJ: "Sometimes I'll use chocolate or cookies, but what I really like are hugs from people I love."

DK: "When I need comfort, I usually take a nap. But sometimes I'll have a cup of hot chocolate."

JS: "I never use food to comfort myself. I work out."

KK: "I never turn to food when I'm stressed. Actually I lose my appetite if I'm under a lot of pressure. I like to talk or get a massage, even just a foot massage."

MM: "I sometimes will turn to pasta or ice cream. If I do, I just accept the moment; I don't feel guilty. More often I use books, TV, crossword puzzles, or magazines."

As you can see, even naturally slim people find themselves needing to escape from the pressures of everyday life. They choose to spend the time doing something relaxing or nurturing for themselves. They enjoy just being with themselves and nurture themselves with tea, rest, books, exercise, and naps rather than food.

Being Slim Does Not Mean Being Perfect

Naturally slim people talk lovingly of their favorite restaurant, the wonderful pumpkin pie that their aunt Sarah makes, which they can't resist, and their favorite flavor of ice cream. As an ex–chronic dieter I was amazed by this. I used to think that naturally slim people viewed food strictly as sustenance, that eating was something they reluctantly participated in to keep their body running as they fulfilled some greater purpose. Finding out that having favorite foods that were not particularly nutritious and occasionally overeating was normal for slim people took a big load off my mind. This whole process appears much more feasible when we realize that we don't have to eat "perfectly" for the rest of our lives.

The whole process of becoming healthy is not an all-or-nothing proposition. Each small step that we take in a positive direction is just that—a step in a positive direction! Each time we take a step in a negative direction it is an opportunity to learn. The key to health, happiness, and indeed optimal body weight is not to eliminate all the negatives and do only the positive. The key is recognizing that life is full of both, the yin and the yang, the black and the white, the light and the dark. It is contrast that gives depth and meaning to our existence. When you come to see your "mistakes" as just as valuable as your progress, you are fully involved in determining the course of your life.

Balance is what we desire—balance in eating and hungering, balance in moving and resting, balance in stretching our minds and just being. Balance does not mean standing still but refers to a dynamic equilibrium where we are constantly moving between opposite sides, never tarrying too long on one side or the other and always moving closer to the center.

Opportunities for Growth

Awareness

- Allow yourself to get hungry. What does it feel like? Using the Hunger-Satisfaction Scale in Figure 2, what sensations do you have at −1, −3, −5? How do you eat at each of these levels? Is it more difficult to eat slowly and stop if you start at −5 instead of −2?

- Track your hunger signals for several days. If you are very busy, do you notice your hunger signals? When it is lunchtime, are you hungry at all? Notice when you get hungry and how hungry you get (use the scale provided). If you eat, how long does it satisfy you?

- Put a sign in your kitchen that asks, "Why are you here?" If you find yourself foraging, check yourself for nutrient hunger. What did you have for your last several meals? Are you short on water? Protein? Fresh fruit? Fresh vegetables? Have you been keeping your fat grams so low you're craving fat? If it's not nutrient hunger, is it psychological hunger? Even if you don't want to think about it now, at least take the time to think about it after you eat instead of just feeling guilty.

Introspection

- When your hunger is not physically or nutritionally based, recognize this. Be OK with it. Say, "I realize that I am eating at this moment for emotional reasons, and I promise myself that I'll find out why." Keep your commitment to yourself. What emotional hole are you trying to fill up with the cookies, chips, or ice cream that you chose?

- Many people identify loneliness as one of the reasons they eat. You can't be lonely unless you do not like the person you are alone with. Do you like the person you are alone with—yourself?

Old Beliefs to Let Go

- I'm always hungry.

- If I allow myself to get hungry, I'll eat everything in sight.

- I'm so fat I should never be hungry.

- Food is a good substitute for love.

New Beliefs to Embrace

- It is natural to feel hungry.

- I easily recognize the difference between my physical and emotional hungers.

- I eat food only when I'm physically hungry.

- I nurture myself with love and comfort when I am emotionally hungry.

Vividly Imagine

- Imagine yourself in the last emotional state where you turned to food, or make up such a situation. Now take yourself through that situation, feel the feelings—the sadness or loneliness or whatever they were—and see yourself in the kitchen reaching for that food. Now imagine yourself changing your mind. Give yourself permission to do anything you desire for comfort instead of eating—a manicure, a trip to the Bahamas, a hug from your mother. Then give yourself that comfort. Enjoy yourself and feel the distressing feelings melt away.

Patterns for Action

- Prepare a list of your personal comfort activities that can begin to take the place of food, and post it in the kitchen. When you are ready, begin to choose them in times of emotional stress.

- Eat when you are physically hungry. Be prepared by having nutritious snacks available. Set aside a certain number of days as a trial period to get the hang of it. The goal is eventually to eat *only* when you are physically hungry. Ignore artificial designations of lunchtime, dinnertime, coffee break, etc. Listen to your body, not the clock or someone else's body.

- Ease yourself out of nighttime eating so you can feel hungry for breakfast in the morning.

- Take the time to prepare a balanced snack—one that contains protein, carbohydrate, and fat (see Chapter 18)—to take to work or keep in the car in case you get hungry.

Additional Reading

Dufty, William. *Sugar Blues*. Radnor: Chilton Books, 1975.

Louden, Jennifer. *The Woman's Comfort Book*. San Francisco: HarperCollins, 1992.

Munter, Carol, and Jane Hirschman. *Overcoming Overeating*. New York: Fawcett Columbine, 1989.

Strauss, Steven C., M.D., and Gail North. *Body Signal Secrets*. Emmaus, PA: Rodale Press, 1991.

Triboli, Evelyn, M.S., R.D., and Elyse Resch, M.S., R.D. *Intuitive Eating*. New York: St. Martin's Press, 1995.

NINE

Habit 6: Be a Picky Eater

Being picky about what you eat is a sign of self-respect. Not only is it OK to be picky about what you eat, but it is also essential to the process of becoming naturally slim.

IT WAS A BALMY October day. I positioned myself strategically on the terrace of a popular restaurant to observe corporate lunchtime. Men and women arrived in groups of two or more, well dressed and ready to take a break from their routines. It was a time to refresh physically and mentally. My mission: to observe their eating patterns. I selected two women whose table was close enough to me that I could observe them without being too obtrusive. One of the women was considerably fatter than the other; we'll call her Jane. The slender woman we'll call Pat. As I watched the lunchtime scenario unfold, I was forced to recall the characters in the nursery rhyme "Jack Sprat." However, a kind of role reversal appeared to be going on as I recalled the part of the poem that goes "Jack Sprat could eat no fat, his wife could eat no lean." In this instance the overweight woman was eating what might be considered "lean," and the slim woman was eating what might be considered "fat." Even more remarkable than what was on their plates, though, was the way they ate their food.

Jane had gone to the salad bar and had a platter heaped with greens and a bit of potato salad and macaroni salad. Her dressing was thick and creamy but on the side, two small plastic cups of it. She also had a muffin and butter and a large diet soda. Pat ordered a chicken breast with pasta Alfredo, a salad, and a piece of pie. I looked at my watch as they began eating and then took in the entire experience of what was to be a classic lunch shared by a chronic dieter (Jane) and a naturally slim person (Pat).

Jane talked almost incessantly during the meal. She took both containers of dressing and drizzled them over her salad. She took large bites of lettuce and appeared famished as she consumed the entire platter of salad in 15 minutes. Pat, on the other hand, appeared to be listening to Jane and offering comments at intervals. However, it was clear that she was paying close attention to her meal at the same time. She carefully poured a bit of salad dressing on her salad and ate a few bites. Then she switched to her main course, discreetly dissecting the sauce-laden skin from the chicken. Next she scraped a bit of the Alfredo sauce off the pasta to the side of her plate and began to cut the chicken into tiny bite-size pieces. She ate slowly, chewing each bite thoroughly, occasionally eating some salad in between. After 20 minutes she had eaten two-thirds of her salad, two-thirds of her chicken, and a third to half of the pasta and sauce. She pushed the plate aside and asked for some coffee to go with her dessert. Jane said she was not having dessert, though she had finished the large blueberry muffin with butter on it. Jane sipped her diet pop and talked while she waited for Pat to eat dessert. Pat ate three bites of pie, declared the crust soggy, and finished her coffee. The meal was officially over for Pat in 25 minutes.

Who do you think had the healthier lunch? Who was more satisfied by what she ate? Who left the table feeling deprived?

Forget what your mother told you. It is OK to be a picky eater. Not only is it OK, but it is necessary and desirable to reach your optimal body weight. The naturally slim people we interviewed had a lot to say about what they will and will not eat. They never eat what they don't like, even if someone's feelings might be hurt. They simply are unable to violate their body's natural wisdom, which is true self-love. They like their hot foods hot, their cold foods cold, and when food loses its proper temperature, they just don't eat it. Crisp things should be crisp, and fresh things fresh. They scrape off sauces they don't like no matter who is watching, and if they order a piece of chocolate cake and want only a bite, they eat the bite and leave the rest. They feel absolutely no need to clean their plate or to eat for all the starving children anywhere.

Naturally slim people enjoy a wide variety of foods and enjoy trying new foods but deplore having food foisted on them when they are not hungry. Also, the people we interviewed did not care much for fast food and never ate meals while driving in a car. If a meal at a restaurant was not hot or was cooked incorrectly, they would send it back. If they tried a new dish and found they really didn't care for it, they would leave it and focus on other parts of the meal to satisfy their hunger. If they were in the mood for dessert, they would have a light meal and a whole dessert, or they would order just dessert, or they would have a whole dinner, eat two bites of dessert, and leave the rest. Sweets were not a big issue with naturally slim people, for they were not considered "bad" foods and therefore had no more appeal than anything else they might have an occasional taste for.

Being Picky Is Not Bad

Being a picky eater has a negative connotation in some people's eyes. As children, our parents disdained the picky eater, the one who did not like string beans, would not eat leftovers, or would not finish his soup unless it was warmed up again. As adults we have seen a picky eater send his steak back three times to get the restaurant kitchen to cook it to his satisfaction. We may feel that we are catering to whims and spoiling a child who is picky, or we may feel embarrassed by a friend who sends things back at a restaurant. If you've felt this way, ask yourself why. If a child takes at least two or three bites of a food on her plate and genuinely dislikes it, should we force her to eat the rest? Should we bring out the plate of offending food every time the child is hungry for the next four days, because if she is *really* hungry she'll eat it? When eating out and paying sometimes exorbitant amounts of money for a meal, shouldn't we feel OK about requesting that it be done to our satisfaction? Isn't that the idea of eating out? Yes, there is a fine line between being picky and being obnoxious and I'm sure we have all known both adults and children who have crossed that line. However, the innate desire to give ourselves pleasure by eating foods that we like and foods that are prepared well is an instinct worth preserving.

How Often Do You Compromise on What You Really Want to Eat?

When you are embarrassed by someone who politely sends back a meal at a restaurant, is it because you wouldn't have the guts to do it yourself? Would you rather be quiet and eat what is on your plate, like it or not, because you don't want to suffer the disapproving glance of a friend or a waiter? Do you go and eat fast food with the rest of the office even though you would really like a bowl of hot soup and some fresh bread? How often do you compromise and eat something you don't care for that much, just because it is easier? Giving up your innate pickiness can contribute to becoming overweight. When you continuously compromise your eating desires and eat what is available, what everyone else is eating, or what your mother wants you to, you eat less-than-satisfying meals. When your meals aren't satisfying, you search elsewhere for that satisfaction by eating more, eating secretly, or eating high-fat, high-sugar foods in rebellion, all of which are very self-defeating ways to exert your independence.

Begin to eat exactly what you like. Be OK eating dessert instead of a meal; be OK turning down Mother's meat loaf or just pushing it around on your plate. Take the time to pack yourself exactly what you would like for lunch and then go along with your friends to eat and socialize no matter where they choose to go. Stop and pick up what you want to eat and meet the others wherever they are going. Tell them you have food allergies or whatever you need to say to be comfortable with what you are doing. But the truth is you are doing it for yourself because you care about yourself. You care enough to be picky about what you eat.

Tune In to Your Body Before You Tune In to Your Refrigerator

Suppose you're at home and, because you have been practicing tuning in to your hunger signals, you are able to determine that, yes, indeed, you are hungry. The next step you probably take is to go into the kitchen and see what is available. We would like you to rethink that step. Before you go see what's available, listen to your body and see if you can determine what it wants to eat. This is important especially in the beginning stages of becoming naturally slim because you may not have begun to stock your kitchen with a wide variety of foods. After you decide what you really want and need to eat, go to the kitchen and see if you have it. If not, go out and get exactly what you want. I know this may seem a bit extreme, but in the beginning of this process of getting to know and respect your body, following through on your intuition builds trust. Once you start keeping a wider variety of foods in your house, you will find you do not need to go out that often. The idea is to be totally self-referred when choosing what to eat. When you limit yourself to what is in your refrigerator, you compromise your choices.

The "Maybe the Next Bite Will Be Better" Syndrome

Sitting in my favorite restaurant one Friday evening, I could hardly wait until dessert because they serve the best bread pudding with hot caramel sauce I have ever tasted. After dinner I ordered my dessert, and when it arrived I took a very small forkful, ready to savor every morsel. It was not at all what I remembered. It lacked sweetness, it was a little cold, and the edges were crusty. Not at all what I expected, so I took another bite. It tasted the same, less than good. So I had another bite and complained to my husband, "Boy, this bread pudding isn't at all what I remember." When I asked if they had changed the recipe, they said no. I ate another bite and another, somehow thinking if I kept eating it would eventually fulfill my expectations. There I was, 15 minutes and 400 calories later, still wanting a good dish of bread pudding. If I had just valued myself and my first impression, I could have asked for another piece or chosen another dessert. Mostly, I needed to realize that I enjoy good bread pudding and don't need to wait until once every six months to get some. Maybe then the disappointment over a single dessert would not have been so monumental that I felt driven to finish it with little satisfaction.

Buy foods that you like even if your family doesn't and keep them in the house. You deserve fresh food. You deserve to have weird spices and hot peppers and fresh bread. If you are going to eat chocolate, buy the best, eat it slowly, and enjoy the quality. The more you deny yourself certain foods, the more you will crave them. The more you buy cheap substitutes or fat-free substitutes for your favorite foods, the more you will experience the bite-after-bite-after-bite syndrome that I just described. A low-fat substitute can send you on a fattening search for satisfaction, a satisfaction that can't be found unless you allow yourself to buy and eat the real thing.

Many people feel that if they consider food an enemy and shopping and cooking to be chores, they will be able to keep their weight down. Actually the opposite is true. The less picky we are about our food, the less shopping for fresh produce that we do, and the less cooking and more convenience foods we use, the poorer our nutritional intake is. When our nutritional intake is poor, we develop food cravings and tend to forage more, eating even though we are not hungry because we are searching for certain nutrients. If you do see food as the enemy and shopping as a chore, these are ingrained subconscious beliefs that need to be changed, or you will never allow yourself to do anything different.

How sad that we abuse our bodies, feeding them lukewarm food, stale leftovers, and greasy drive-through because we don't love ourselves enough to take the time and energy to get the good wholesome food our bodies really desire. When you are hungry, be picky about what you eat. When you honor yourself and your preferences, you reinforce trust and love for your body. Naturally slim people are very picky about what they eat, and they can be so without being socially obnoxious. Devouring the first food you happen to see when hungry shows little respect for the process of nourishing your body and is a step away from the health and slimness you say you so desperately desire.

Opportunities for Growth

Awareness

- Look in your refrigerator and cabinets. Do you see a wide variety of foods? Do you have some of your favorite foods, healthy and not so healthy, on hand? Do you have fresh fruits and vegetables in the house? Do you have quick protein pick-me-ups on hand (cheese, nuts, meats, fish, legumes)?

- Observe your attitudes about and approach to shopping. Do you hate shopping? Do you take the time to plan meals and shop for them? Do you run into and out of the grocery store, grabbing whatever you see as fast as you can? Do you read labels so that you know what you're really eating?

- Listen to what your body says it wants to eat. The next time you are hungry, before you decide what to eat, sit quietly with yourself in whole-brain posture (see Chapter 17) and ask yourself, "If I could have any combination of food in the world, what would truly nourish me right now?"

- Observe your actions concerning meal selection. Did you take the time to listen to your body? If you took the time, did you honor your body's request? If you didn't, what kept you from honoring it?

- Observe yourself choosing meals and eating them. Did you listen to your body before you chose the meal? Did you pay attention to what you were eating and how it was prepared? Was it the proper temperature and texture, seasoned as you like? Did it have too much or too little sauce or crunch, or was it lumpy when you like it smooth? If it wasn't the way you like it, did you fix it to your liking? Or did you eat it anyway?

- Feel the texture and taste of your food. Do you like it? After you swallow several bites, how does it sit in your stomach? Does it feel heavy, greasy, light, satisfying?

- As often as possible experience the absolute joy and pleasure of being hungry and eating exactly what your body wants.

Introspection

- Are you taking the time to become aware of yourself and what you think and do concerning shopping for, choosing, and eating food?

- What you eat is between you and your body. Are you consulting your body? Are you eating certain foods at certain times based on someone else's preferences or just to "keep the peace"?

- Are you constantly compromising your preferences when it comes to your choice of foods and eating?

- Do you continue eating even after you've determined an item does not taste very good or is not what you expected?

Old Beliefs to Let Go

- I hate food shopping.

- I don't have time to talk to my body every time I eat.

- If I'm picky about what I eat, people won't like it.

- Leaving food on my plate is a waste of food and money.

- If I ask my body what it wants to eat, it will only want sweets and fats and other "bad" foods.

- Keeping the peace at the table is more important than my food preferences.

New Beliefs to Embrace

- Food shopping is an enjoyable part of becoming a naturally slim person.

- I always consult my body's needs when choosing what to eat.

- I love myself; therefore I am picky about the food I eat.

- Leaving food on my plate when I'm satisfied is a loving gesture of health.

- My body calls for healthy, natural foods, and I hear its messages clearly.

- My food preferences are important to me.

- I am unconcerned about what other people think of my eating habits.

Vividly Imagine

- Read the "New Beliefs" section again. This time highlight words that do not create a clear picture in your mind—words such as *picky, preferences, enjoyable, healthy*. Just because you use them all the time does not mean you necessarily have a clear picture about them, especially in the context of food, eating, and body image. Now create a vivid image in your mind of yourself as a picky shopper and then a picky eater. Incorporate the new beliefs that you want to embrace. Use the senses of sight, sound, taste, touch, and smell to make the image vivid. See yourself in all sorts of situations where you might choose to be a picky eater to enhance your health and natural slimness, and then add in your other senses. What would you say? What would other people say about you? Feel the pleasure it brings to take care of yourself and your health when you shop and eat this way. Fill in as many details as possible—the more the better.

Patterns for Action

- When you find yourself in some sort of distracted thinking, worrying, or other nongrowth state of mind, recall your mental image and the pleasure it gives you. Do this as often as you wish.

- Look deep into your own eyes in the mirror and affirm the new beliefs listed earlier. With each affirmation, recall the part of your vivid image that portrays that belief in action. Do this once a day. If you can't get yourself to do this, don't judge yourself and don't quit. Choose another activity that focuses on increasing your health and self-esteem.

- When you are ready, begin the process of being picky when you shop, cook, and eat. Take it one day, one meal, one bite at a time.

Additional Reading

David, Marc. *Nourishing Wisdom*. New York: Bell Tower, 1991.
Hirschman, Jane, and Lela Zaphiropoulos. *Solving Your Child's Eating Problems*. New York: Fawcett Columbine, 1985.
Munter, Carol, and Jane Hirschman. *Overcoming Overeating*. New York: Fawcett Columbine, 1989.

Habit 7: Savor Your Eating Experiences

Savoring is an art that can enhance your entire life. The practice of slowing down, appreciating small things, and immersing yourself in the present increases your ability to derive satisfaction from every life experience, including the experience of eating.

SITTING ON A wooden bench, beside a crab apple tree laden with blossoms, Sharon reached into a rumpled brown paper bag and pulled out her lunch. She always enjoyed her early-morning ritual of choosing what she wanted for lunch and carefully wrapping it in plastic. She was thinking of getting one of those insulated lunch boxes with the blue plastic thing you could freeze, but she hadn't quite gotten around to it. Today it was Swiss cheese on rye, an apple, and a handful of sunflower seeds. After eyeing the food she had chosen, she decided to save the sunflower seeds for later and placed them back in the bag on the bench next to her. She polished the apple on her shirt and carefully opened the plastic wrap on the sandwich. She picked up one half of the sandwich and held it up to her nose. Next she lifted up the top piece of bread and rearranged the cheese so that she would get a bite of cheese with every bite of bread.

Lifting the sandwich to her mouth, she sank her teeth right into the center of the longest side, the one without the crust. The spicy dryness of the bread collapsed into the moistness of the cheese, and the bite landed on her tongue. As she pushed it around between tongue and teeth, the contrast of the rough dry bread and the cool smooth cheese delighted her taste buds. Salty, sour, pungent, sweet, they exploded sometimes singly and sometimes all at once. Slowly as she chewed, the tastes blended together into a smooth, sweet liquid, which she swallowed. A very soft "mmmmm" escaped her lips. I was sooo hungry, she thought, as well as, This tastes soooo good. She took a deep breath of the spring air, and the corners of her mouth turned up in a contented smile. She examined the new shape of her sandwich and began the process again, savoring every moment.

Didn't Sharon's mother tell her not to play with her food? Wasn't she told to "stop dawdling and hurry up and eat"? Didn't her school have 20-minute lunch breaks where you spent 10 minutes in line waiting to get your food? Maybe, maybe not. Whatever her background, she believes what we all need to believe to unleash our naturally slim instincts: Eating is meant to be enjoyed, and you are worthy of the time it takes to eat every meal with joy and respect for your body. This does not mean that eating should be your only joy in life. If it is, that may be the reason you are overweight. Eating and satisfying hunger is meant to be one of the joys of life. However, there are thousands of joys in our lives if we know how to look for them and, even more important, how to savor and enjoy them.

Naturally Slim People Savor Their Food

Food is meant to be flavorful, spicy, savory, brightly colored, a variety of temperatures and textures, fun, enjoyable, and satisfying. When was the last time you had a meal that was all those things? Last month at a restaurant? No wonder you overate; the experience was probably so grand that you didn't want it to stop! At our command post as observers of naturally slim people we were routinely mesmerized by the meticulousness with which they ate their meals. They were totally engrossed in their food. Even when sharing a meal with another person, as soon as the food was served their participation in the conversation at the table decreased. Their eyes focused on their plates, they looked at their food, maybe even turned the plate around, pushed certain foods to the side that they didn't plan to eat, and sniffed the aroma of each and every food. The subjects we observed always tasted their food before adding salt or pepper or other condiments.

Perhaps the most consistent observation we made of naturally slim people was that they took tiny bites, left their fork empty, and chewed a very long time. Their meals ranged in length from 20 to 45 minutes. Several diets on the market address the concept of eating more slowly by telling dieters to take bites the size of a pea, put the fork down between bites, and chew each bite 25 times. The problem with this well-meaning advice is that it requires you to follow someone else's directions rather than listen to your own body. Even more important, it causes you to miss the entire experience of eating because you're too busy counting. These directives can work quite well if you use them once in a while as an exercise in awareness, but forcing yourself to do them at every single meal to lose weight is an exercise in futility.

A Recipe for Savoring

Once you have decided that you are hungry, and have chosen exactly what your body wants to eat, find a relaxing spot, stop talking, turn off the TV, and enjoy.

The Setting

Whenever you have the opportunity, exert your right to choose the setting in which you eat. Choosing a setting that is pleasing to the eye and relaxing to the mind can provide you with mental and spiritual nourishment along with your primary objective, physical nourishment. Eating outdoors can be particularly renewing. Sitting in a park surrounded by greenery, your body picks up the energy and the oxygen of being surrounded by living things. Eating outside at a drive-through, where your table is sitting on a concrete slab right next to trucks and cars spewing out exhaust fumes, will not be a very nourishing experience. Many of us pass our days without getting a ray of sunshine or a breath of fresh air. We go from house to car to office to car to restaurant to car to office to car to home. It is not just a myth that fresh air and sunshine are essential to health. They are cheap and readily available; include some in your next snack or meal.

The Look

Slow down and purposefully look at what is on your plate. Foods with a variety of colors and textures are satisfying to our sense of beauty and balance. Chefs spend hours designing the eye appeal of their dishes because when food looks good it feeds more than the body; it feeds the spirit, too. A little piece of parsley or an orange slice can turn "just lunch" into a dining experience.

After appreciating the look of your meal, begin to imagine the taste of each food and how it will feel in your mouth. Think about which part of the meal you want to be sure to have room for and make a mental note of it. If you imagine eating one of the foods and it no longer appeals to you, mentally or physically put it over to the side of the plate. Check in with your stomach, note how hungry you are, and estimate how much food you need to eat. You can even mark your servings with a fork or knife to remind yourself of the amount that you thought would satisfy your current level of hunger. When you have eaten to the lines, stop and reevaluate your hunger.

The Sniff

Our sense of smell is meant to protect us as well as give us pleasure. We can smell smoke before we see it or know that something is rancid before we consume it and in this way ensure our physical safety. Smell is also an integral part of the eating experience. As we lift a fork to our mouth, by default we smell our food. If we add purpose to that act and notice and register those smells, we can add to the satisfaction of our eating experiences. Aromas stimulate specific areas of our brain. Not only do they bring forward memories associated with a particular smell, but they also can be used to reduce stress, produce energy, facilitate sleep, and more, depending on the area of the brain they stimulate. This principle is the foundation for aromatherapy, the therapeutic use of aromas for healing. Also, smell is an integral part of taste. Food can often seem tasteless when our nose is stuffed up and our appetite tends to wane. Note the aroma of each food on your plate or each ingredient in your sandwich. Become aware of whether it enhances the pleasure of your meal. Also, notice if it stimulates any thoughts or feelings or memories.

The Bite

The smaller the bite you take, the more the surface area of your food can come in contact with your taste buds. It also allows for an increased saliva-to-food ratio, which improves digestion and absorption of nutrients. In other words, eating smaller bites allows you to be better nourished by what you eat than with large bites. Big bites are difficult to savor, and they can also hide small inedible things such as pebbles that should have been picked out of dried beans or woody stems that should have been trimmed from herbs or worse—I once almost swallowed a small screw that was hidden in a giant bite of mashed potatoes! In the worst-case scenario large bites (or talking while eating) can cause you to choke.

Remember, eating, like the rest of life, is a process. The objective of the process is to take a break from whatever you are doing and nourish yourself. The objective is not to get to the end as soon as possible. Eating one peanut at a time instead of a handful or filling your fork half full instead of heaping it is not meant to deprive you of anything. You can still eat the entire serving.

Then again, you may not need to, because you have given your-self the experience of savoring and enjoying many bites and you are eating slowly enough that your brain has the time to send you appropriate satisfaction signals before you overeat.

The Taste

Some of you have been exposed to more tastes than others. Some of you grew up on meat, potatoes, and corn, and therefore any-thing that does not taste like meat, potatoes, and corn strikes fear in your heart or puts disgust on your face. The taste of food can stimulate your metabolism and your digestion. It can also give you pleasure. Eating bland foods with little variation in taste con-tributes to inattentiveness at meals and overeating. Face it, it is hard to ignore a bowl of red-hot chili! Also, our so-called crav-ings for salt or sweet may in fact be cravings to have our taste buds stimulated, yet because we are mostly familiar with sweet and salt we go for those rather than other tastes.

Ayurveda, a traditional Eastern philosophy of health, states that six tastes are part of a healthy diet and that we should attempt to include each one in our meals:

1. Bitter—bitter greens, endive, romaine, spinach, tonic water

2. Sweet—pasta, milk, honey, rice, cream, butter, sugar, wheat

3. Sour—lemons, cheese, yogurt, plums, vinegar

4. Salty—any food with salt added

5. Pungent—ginger, chili peppers, cayenne

6. Astringent—beans, lentils, apples, pears, cabbage, pomegranates

Become aware of the tastes in your meals. Avoid judgments such as "This tastes good" or "This tastes bad." Instead of judg-ing, be aware of whether your eating experiences have a variety of quality tastes. Consider expanding your spice cabinet. If you're having something sweet and sour like cottage cheese, add some curry powder or some apple slices and expand the taste. Adding a variety of tastes to your meals increases satisfaction and decreases cravings.

If you find there are certain tastes that you absolutely cannot tolerate, such as hot foods or sour foods, ask yourself what may have caused your aversion to this taste. I discovered the reason that I dislike foods with red pepper in them when a childhood memory came to me. In our house, a sprinkle of red pepper on the tongue was the consequence for lying or using bad language. With that type of association, no wonder I don't like red pepper! Maybe you ate a whole jar of pickles and made yourself sick one time, and you can't stand the taste of anything sour. These negative associations with certain foods can be reversed, as you'll learn in Chapter 17.

The Temperature

Eating foods at a pleasant temperature increases the satisfaction of a meal. If a food is cold and the fat is congealing around it, don't eat it. If it's too hot or too cold, warm it or let it sit and cool down. You have the time, and you deserve to have maximum enjoyment from your food.

The Texture

Have you ever wondered why they take the same flour and eggs used for good old spaghetti and turn them into shells, wagon wheels, rotini, radiatore, and other fanciful shapes? Eye appeal is one reason, but the most important is so you can play with them with your tongue! It is OK to play with your food—in fact we recommend it. Remember that overwhelming urge you had as a child to suck each strand of spaghetti into your mouth instead of using your fork? Well, with short pasta you can play with it with your tongue and no one will even notice. Feel the twists and turns of the noodles. Put a wagon wheel on the end of your tongue. Taste which pasta shapes hold more sauce. Experiment with eating your pasta al dente, with a little crunch, instead of soft and mushy. Try whole-grain pasta of wheat, quinoa, or spelt. They are much more nutritious than pasta made of white flour and have a hearty texture.

Feel the crispness, hear the crunch, slide the smoothness over your tongue, and catch it on your tonsils. Have fun and pay attention to texture. Take a texture inventory of your meals. If a meal consists of creamed soup, mashed potatoes, whipped squash, some sort of meat, and white bread, you may end up experiencing texture deprivation. That's when you head for the potato chips— because you just need to crunch. Increasing the variety of textures in your meals increases satisfaction and decreases cravings.

The Chew

We were given teeth for a reason: to bite, tear, and chew our food. Chewing gives us a sense of satisfaction in and of itself. It is a powerful muscular motion that can defuse anger and frustration as well as help our bodies with digestion. It is no wonder that in this high-stress world people chew gum, chew tobacco, chew their nails . . . and if that's not enough, they turn to pretzels, potato chips, and corn chips to bite down and hear that satisfying crunch! If we take the time to be aware of our feelings, and honor them (see Chapter 8), maybe we won't have the overwhelming desire to keep our jaws clenched on chips. If we chew our food more every time we eat, instead of gulping it in and sliding it down our throats with as few chews as possible, we will eat less and allow our digestion to work properly. Our stomach was not meant to receive huge chunks of food, or we would have been given a second stomach. We are meant to chew our food into a very digestible liquid and in that way put less stress on our gastrointestinal tracts.

The Swallow

Swallowing is a voluntary act. Food does not swallow itself. Small bites that are chewed well allow swallowing to be a pleasant experience. Large bites poorly chewed may cause you to feel a lump in your throat or your chest. Take your time and chew so that your food can properly nourish you. If you are aware that swallowing is a voluntary act, you won't be hurried by the fact that you already filled your fork for the next bite. Sometimes we get caught in a vicious cycle of hurried eating that is driven by the fact that we fill our forks for the next bite as soon as they are empty.

I remember distinctly how I used to take a bite, begin to chew, and then look around my plate and choose the next bite— all the while chewing and not paying any attention to what was in my mouth. The visual cue of the full fork would cause me to chew and swallow even faster to prepare for the bite that was forked and ready to go. This is a great example of focusing so intently on the future that we forget to enjoy the present. After the swallow comes the satisfaction we feel as the food hits the stomach and begins to fill the emptiness of our hunger. The entire next chapter is devoted to satisfaction.

In eating, just as in life, we often focus so intently on the future that we forget to enjoy the present. If we savor every present moment of our eating and our life, we won't need a lump of food stuck in our throat or an extra 50 pounds of fat to wake us up and get our attention. Don't count the number of times you chew each bite; don't even put your fork down between bites. Just pay attention; become aware of all the possibilities each bite of food has to offer and savor them all. As you master the art of savoring your food, begin to savor other aspects of your life: work, play, vacation, a sunset, a thunderstorm, friends, children, the book you're reading, or even the dishes you are washing.

Opportunities for Growth

Awareness

- Observe yourself eating meals and snacks. How fast do you eat? Do you finish without even having noticed what you are eating? Do you talk, watch TV, or read while eating? Do you load up your fork for the next bite when you haven't finished chewing the first? When you swallow, is your food chewed well? Is it smooth and liquid?

- Take one chocolate kiss and follow the recipe for savoring. Don't even chew it. Suck on it and play with it in your mouth until it is melted and gone. If you ate each bite of chocolate that way, do you think you would overindulge? Try the exercise with a single grape, rolling it around whole in your mouth until you can't resist biting into it and tasting the sweet liquid. Also try a raisin or a peanut.

Introspection

- When you are eating, are you present with your food and your body? Or are your mind and your attention miles away? Eating is a celebration and renewal of your life energy. If you give eating the respect it deserves, your food will give you the nourishment you deserve.

- Are you always in a hurry? Is time still an issue for you? If so, return again to Habit 1 on life priorities and Habit 2 on self-love. If health is a life priority and you care about yourself, you will find the time.

Beliefs to Let Go

- I don't have the time to savor meals.

- It's what I eat, not how I eat, that makes me fat.

- If I enjoy the food I'm eating, I'll eat too much.

- If I pay attention to my food, I'll feel guilty because I shouldn't be eating it.

Beliefs to Embrace

- I eat slowly and enjoy my food as a celebration of life.

- Savoring my food helps me reach my naturally slim state of health.

- I eat small amounts of nutritious food, and I thoroughly enjoy every bite.

- I lovingly pay attention to the food I am eating.

Vividly Imagine

- In your mind, select the most wonderful meal you can imagine. Now imagine yourself savoring every bite of that meal using the recipe for savoring in this chapter. Allow yourself to smell the smells, taste the tastes, feel the temperatures and textures. Experience the sensory satisfaction and notice how few bites it takes to satisfy your hunger when you eat like this.

Patterns for Action

- Use the recipe for savoring anytime anywhere you are eating, whether it is dinner in a restaurant or popcorn in a theater. Savor as many eating experiences as possible until savoring becomes an automatic part of your eating habits.

Additional Reading

Chopra, Deepak, M.D. *Creating Health.* Boston: Houghton Mifflin, 1987 (Chapter 26).

Chopra, Deepak, M.D. *Perfect Weight.* New York: Harmony Books, 1994.

ELEVEN

Habit 8: Feel Satisfied Instead of Full

Every time you eat according to your natural instincts, it is an act of love and respect. When you begin to recognize your body's needs and take the utmost care in satisfying them, the feelings of self-connectedness can be awesome.

THE MERE CONTEMPLATION of the dictionary definition for satisfaction causes me to take a deep breath and sigh. *Satisfaction* is a wonderful word, and it is a wonderful feeling. All of the anxiety we have attached to food and eating has caused us to forget the simple joys of feeling hungry and satisfying our need for food. Clear your head, take a deep breath, and read this definition: *Satisfaction is the act of fully gratifying wants, desires, and wishes, putting an end to needs or wants.* It is gratification. It is demands fully met. It is the condition of being pleased, content, and fulfilled. Doesn't that sound great? Wouldn't that feel great? It can be yours every time you eat, if you desire.

The skills presented in the preceding three chapters—eating only when you're hungry, being picky about what you eat, and savoring your food—all contribute to your sense of satisfaction.

It is difficult to feel satisfied if you are eating when you are not even hungry, if you are eating what's available instead of what you really want, and if you are eating rapidly with little attention to the experience. Knowing what satisfies you in a meal and putting down your fork when you are satisfied is one of the most important skills you can develop.

We asked naturally slim people to describe the feeling they get when they know it is time to stop eating. Here are some of the answers we received: "I don't know; I just know." "I don't know for sure, but I hate feeling full or sluggish, so I rarely eat to that point, except maybe at Thanksgiving." I know it's time to stop eating when "I'm no longer hungry," "I've had enough and I'm ready to move on," "I feel light, energized," "The food no longer tastes as good as it did; it doesn't appeal to me any longer," "I feel comfortably full, not stuffed," "I feel satisfied; I don't need anymore." You may notice that none of the answers were "When my plate is empty," "When I've finished dessert," or "When my belt feels tight." Naturally slim people stop eating when their need for nourishment is satisfied, whether the "meal" is crackers and cheese or a seven-course dinner at a five-star restaurant.

Self-Referred Versus Other-Referred

The decision to stop eating must be self-referred just as the decision to start eating must be self-referred. You must pay attention to your self and your body when you make the decision, not to what someone else is doing or what someone else tells you to do. Your cues, or signals to start and stop eating, must come from inside you. If you stop eating according to external cues, signals outside yourself, you may stop before you are satisfied or you may eat past your sense of satisfaction. Not recognizing when you are satisfied and eating past satisfaction is the sole cause of being overweight in some people.

Typical external cues that overweight people use to stop eating are an empty plate, finishing the last course of a meal or the last chip in the bag, noticing that everyone else at the table has stopped eating, or needing to be somewhere. These cues have nothing to do with satisfaction of the need to nourish themselves! The only internal cue I've heard from overweight clients is, "I quit when I feel full." However, most of the time they say, "I don't even know when I'm full until I am stuffed, and then I feel awful." If you truly love yourself and are in tune with your natural instincts, you will not want to continue eating to the point of pain. This is why we emphasize chapter after chapter that you must work on developing self-love, self-respect, and self-trust the whole time you are working on developing new eating habits. If you do not like or respect yourself, there is no reason for you to change anything that you are doing, whether it is starving, stuffing, bingeing, or purging.

How Do We Sense Satisfaction?

Right next to the hunger or feeding center in the hypothalamus is the satiety center. This center, when stimulated, sends out a signal that directly inhibits the feeding or hunger center so that we no longer have a neurologically based desire to continue eating. The satiety center is stimulated primarily by increased blood sugar and secondarily by increased amino acids (broken-down proteins). As our food is digested, the nutrients enter the bloodstream and the satiety center senses the nutrient levels in our blood. When the nutrient levels in the blood are high enough to satisfy the body's physiological needs, it will send out a "stop" signal to the feeding center.

Your mouth and esophagus serve as monitors of amounts of foods, and when the stomach is distended it also sends signals to inhibit the feeding center. These signals are based purely on the volume of food introduced into the stomach, not on the nutritional quality. This is why we can sometimes eat a meal and feel *full* but not *satisfied*. Our stomach may be distended, but we may not have met our physical, psychological, and nutritional needs, so we remain unsatisfied. In an attempt to become satisfied we continue to eat more of what is in front of us or seek a dessert rather than evaluate specifically what the meal was missing that we might need. This type of eating contributes to our stores of excess body fat. Also, those of you who have developed eating habits based on mealtimes rather than hunger can develop a false sense that you need to eat because you missed a regular mealtime. This is purely a learned response. Rather like Pavlov's dog, we start salivating when the hands on the clock read noon. This learned behavior will diminish over time as you replace eating by the clock with eating according to hunger.

Feeling *full* is an internal cue that reflects the bulk in our stomach. Most of us aren't used to paying attention to how we feel in between "hungry" and "full." In most cases by the time our stomach shouts, "Full!" we have already eaten to the +1 or +2 level on the Hunger-Satisfaction Scale (Chapter 8). When you have hit +1 or +2, you've missed that balanced feeling of satisfaction that naturally slim people use to cue themselves to stop eating. Eating past satisfaction at one meal, coupled with eating the next meal at mealtime instead of when you are hungry, leads to weight gain. Satisfaction is a feeling of balance, of peace, of not hungry and not full but just right—a feeling of being refreshed, "light, energized, and ready to move on." This is what eating is for: to provide you with the energy you need to get on with your life purpose.

Your Metabolic Balance and Your Sense of Satisfaction Are Unique to You

Most of the naturally slim people that we interviewed said they eat three meals and two or three snacks per day. However, some said they eat six small meals or they graze throughout the day. Different body types and different metabolisms may require different time distributions for eating. However, what is apparent in the lifestyles of these naturally slim people is that they do not stick to three meals a day. When you begin to listen closely to your body and eat only when you are hungry and stop eating when you are satisfied, you will find yourself eating smaller amounts of food at more frequent intervals.

Eating small amounts of food at frequent intervals is much healthier than eating three large meals. A large meal often contains more calories than you will need to use in the three to five hours between meals. Unused calories are stored as fat. I know that for some of you, *calorie* is a dirty word. We do not encourage people to count the calories they consume, nor do we encourage people to count the calories they expend. However, we would like you to let go of the notion that calories are "bad." Calories are merely a way scientists have invented to measure the energy potential of food.

We eat food to provide the body with energy. We utilize energy every second of the day—sleeping, meditating, working, playing, thinking, even digesting food. When we consume more calories than we can use, our bodies store them for future use. We can store them as glycogen, a form of stored glucose. However, unless you have been exercising recently, your glycogen storage depots are often full. The alternative storage place is— you guessed it—fat. This is especially true when you eat excess fat calories. Your body finds it very easy to store fat as fat because it is a simple process and takes very little energy. Converting protein and carbohydrates to fat is much more involved.

Your physical body is satisfied with just enough food to meet your energy requirements. If you lead a fairly inactive lifestyle, your energy requirements are small. Balancing your energy intake with your energy use is what will lead to permanent weight loss. I am talking about a natural balance, not an artificial "If I eat a cupcake, I need to run three miles to burn it off" balance. Your body seeks balance naturally. You will be hungry for the exact type and amount of food your body needs to replenish itself and prepare for the afternoon. If you had a sedentary morning and didn't use much energy, you won't be hungry for much food. If you have a very active afternoon, you may be hungry for a larger dinner. This will happen naturally if you pay attention to your body signals. If you have ignored your body's signals for years or decades, it may take a while to get tuned in, but it will happen.

As you experiment with your new eating habits, there may even be a time when you eat so little at a meal that you are hungry in an hour. Don't be dismayed or alarmed when this happens. In any course of learning we often follow the pattern of a pendulum swinging back and forth until it reaches equilibrium. If you are swinging from the position of rarely feeling hungry and eating large meals three times a day, you may very well swing all the way to the opposite extreme of being hungry every hour and eating very tiny meals eight times a day, or grazing. This is OK; you are beginning to pay attention to your body and match feeding times with hunger. Stay on this path of learning and you will find a balance for yourself and your lifestyle.

A report from one of our natural instinctive eaters may be helpful to consider if you are stuck in the phase of eating very small, very frequent meals. A young man we interviewed said when he was really hungry he would usually eat the first two or three bites of his meal rapidly to make the hunger pangs go away. After that he would slow down and enjoy his meal until he no longer was interested in it and felt he had had enough to keep him going until his next break. Many times while I was learning I would stop after those first three bites thinking my hunger was gone and so I had to be satisfied. I found, however, that I would be hungry again in about an hour or even less. Eating every hour is physiologically an OK place to be, but it can be quite inconvenient. I finally realized that those first few bites were just relieving strong hunger pains in my stomach, but they did not meet all of my physiological needs for fuel.

Developing your own sense of hunger and satisfaction comes with paying attention and practice—without judgment. What I did or what you do is not wrong or right; it just is. It is part of learning about yourself. The more you learn about yourself, in body, mind, and spirit, the stronger your loving, caring, health-seeking relationship with yourself will be. Be prepared for your gradual change in eating times. Figure out how you can get a healthy snack or mini-meal at various times during the day. Maybe you will want to pack a little cooler or stock up on some dried soups that can be made with hot water. If you are saying to yourself, "I don't have time for that" or "I can't leave my desk in the middle of the day" or "I don't have a cooler," return to Habit 1 on life priorities and Habit 2 on self-love. If you love yourself and you desire health, you will find the time and the way to take care of yourself and your hungers in a positive way.

What Makes an Eating Experience Satisfying?

Every time you eat, whether you call it a meal or a snack it is an eating experience. Every eating experience is an opportunity to nourish not just your body but your mind and spirit as well. Just taking the time to sit down and eat whatever you have prepared, instead of gulping fast food in the car, is an act of love that nourishes your spirit. The simple act of turning off the television or reducing conversation and really paying attention to what you are putting in your mouth is nourishing and calming to your mind. And of course the actual nutritional content of what you are eating is a gesture of health and kindness to your physical body. These are just a sample of what can be involved in making an eating experience "satisfying" rather than just "filling your stomach." The following topics are meant to take you into the fine art of developing satisfying eating experiences.

Hunger Level

The hungrier you are, the more satisfying a meal can be—up to a point. Eating at a level of 0 to −1 may not be as satisfying as eating at a hunger level of −2 (see Chapter 8 for the Hunger-Satisfaction Scale), especially if you have not allowed yourself to get truly hungry for years. Think of a time when you were out camping or physically active or just very involved in life—so involved that you didn't even realize you were hungry until you were *very* hungry. Can you remember how good that meal tasted and how satisfying it was even though it may have been only freeze-dried beef stew? This is how your level of hunger can contribute to your sense of satisfaction. However, waiting until you are experiencing hunger spasms instead of rumbles or are feeling weak or faint can work the opposite way. People in this severe a state of hunger, even naturally slim people, have a tendency to overeat or to eat rapidly past the sense of satisfaction. Also, waiting until you are in pain before you eat erodes that fledgling sense of trust you have developed between yourself and your body.

Appetite

Eating foods that we have an appetite for increases our satisfaction. However, most of us have distorted our body's natural appetites by feeding it low-quality foods. An appetite for certain foods can be a legitimate message from your body about nutrient needs, or it can just be a "taste" for certain foods that you have connected with the feeling of pleasure. Sweets, chips, chocolate, white flour, and high-fat creamy foods are *learned* appetites. Our body does not have a nutritional need for any of them. (Have you ever heard of a doughnut deficiency?) That does not mean we are saying, "Never eat sweets, chips, or chocolate." That would be asking you to rebel or be a robot, neither of which supports your independence as a natural instinctive eater. What we want to do is increase your awareness. We want you to know what high-quality and low-quality nutrition is and then make your own choices.

Sweets, high-fat foods, chocolate, and chips are nutrient-challenged foods. When you eat a lot of them, you are eating a lot of energy units with very little nutritive value and you will remain hungry for nutrient-dense foods (see Chapter 12). Have them once in a while; they may be filling some psychological need. However, observe yourself when you are eating them. Are you hungry? Are you tense? Are you tired? Do you have anything else in the house to eat? Also look at the amounts you eat; you may well have developed an addiction to them.

Separate from your learned appetites, you may have an appetite for a certain food because it contains a nutrient that your body needs. If you have an appetite for a steak, it may be your body's message that you need protein and iron. Honor that message if at all possible. If you can't get a steak, go for a hamburger. Check in with yourself—you may not even want the bun or side dishes. If you feed your body what it needs and likes instead of what happens to be available or easy to fix, your eating experience will be more satisfying. In our pure unadulterated instinctual state we have desires for healthy nutritious foods, such as vegetables, fruits, whole grains, and beans. However, when you start this natural way of eating you must realize that your natural appetites may be buried and your current appetites may lean toward less-than-healthy foods. Honor these appetites for a while, but during that time expose yourself to new foods. Also immerse your brain in knowledge, thoughts, and beliefs that will support your natural appetites for healthy food. Believe me, we were not born with a natural appetite for chocolate cake and fried chicken.

Attention

Paying attention to what you eat increases the satisfaction of a meal. Naturally slim people do not eat meals in their cars, nor do they watch television during their meals. They really don't care for business lunches and dinners either. Why? Because they don't like to have their attention diverted from their eating experience. How many drive-through meals have you had where you have finished a hamburger and fries without even remembering eating them? When we pay attention to our hunger level, to what we choose for our meals, and then sit down and pay attention to what and how much we are eating, the whole experience of eating changes. We eat more slowly, we chew more thoroughly, we digest our food better, and our meals are more satisfying and more nourishing. If we practice paying attention and being aware, then we can learn to stop eating at the point of satisfaction instead of overeating right past it. Eating with awareness and attention does not mean you have to lock yourself away from everyone and everything when you eat. However, it is a good idea during the learning process to plan to eat several meals a week without any distractions in order to practice the techniques of savoring.

Personally, I often get caught up in the "eat and read" combo meal. I fix myself a nice lunch and then sit down with a book or magazine and read while I eat. The more interesting the reading material, the faster I eat. I can hit the bottom of a bowl of soup in seven minutes and not remember one bite! We are not saying that you can never eat and read or have a drive-through meal. What we are saying is that during this period of retraining your attention you might want to focus totally on your eating experiences and become aware of what and how much you are eating. Add the magazines in later.

Pacing

The amount of time you spend eating your meal or snack is crucial to both your psychological and physical satisfaction with the eating experience. The psychological satisfaction of eating is encouraged when we take a mental break from whatever we are doing to refuel the body. When we allow the mind to relax while refueling the body, we nurture as well as nourish ourselves. In fact doing a short meditation or taking three deep breaths and quieting the mind before a meal may refresh the mind and shift your focus to self-nurturing, loving, and caring for your body. If you are having a business lunch or eating while you're working, not only do you decrease your ability to pay attention to what you are eating, but you also rob yourself of the mental rest you deserve.

Naturally slim people say that they usually spend around 20 minutes eating an average meal. Isn't it interesting that it also takes about 20 minutes from the time you begin eating for the nutrient levels in your blood to become high enough to stimulate your brain's satisfaction center? If you finish a meal in 10 minutes and feel full, 10 minutes later when the nutrients have reached your brain you may feel stuffed. Time some of your typical meals and see how close to 20 minutes you come. I did this a while back while driving in the car eating a large hamburger. Eating that hamburger over 20 minutes felt like an eternity! This is one reason to provide yourself with sit-down, knife-and-fork meals as often as possible.

Convenience foods like sandwiches, hamburgers, fried chicken, and tacos allow you to consume hundreds and hundreds of calories in such a short period of time that it is very easy to eat way past your body's nutritional needs. Sitting down and eating with a knife and fork helps you *pace* your eating. Taking small portions and evaluating your hunger before second servings is also helpful. An empty stomach is about the size of your fist. Although the stomach is meant to expand slightly with meals, and this stretching contributes to satisfaction, it is not meant to stretch to three or four times its size. When you pace yourself and savor (see Chapter 10), it is almost impossible to consume large quantities of food.

Chewing is also an integral part of pacing your meal and assisting your body to digest and assimilate the nutrients you have consumed. Chewing your food and choosing when to swallow it is an entirely voluntary act. Therefore it is within your abilities to speed up or slow down the process. Taking small bites and chewing your food thoroughly allows you to savor your meal and to begin the digestive process by thoroughly mixing the food with the enzymes in your mouth. When food digests well, we get the maximum absorption of nutrients, and the nutrients enter the blood more quickly and easily. This means the brain's satiety center will get a rapid clear message to let you know when to quit eating. Slow down; take your time. Food was meant to be sipped, savored, and enjoyed, not gulped. Doing so will increase your health and decrease your excess fat.

Quality Food

If you follow the first four guidelines using a large candy bar as your meal, you indeed will be satisfied with less candy than usual. The candy will pacify your satisfaction center by raising your blood sugar dramatically. In the long run, however, your physiology will be very dissatisfied because the quality of the fuel you are giving it to run on is very low grade. Eating a meal balanced in protein, carbohydrates, and fats will give your body the ability to provide you with balanced, sustained energy.

Proteins are the building blocks of the body and its immune system. They are also the backbone of the neurological messenger molecules neuropeptides. Neuropeptides provide rapid communication within the brain and between the mind and the body. Carbohydrates are our main energy source, with complex carbohydrates (whole grains, beans, vegetables) providing the best, slow-release source of energy and simple carbohydrates (sweets, white breads, and pastas) providing fast rises and falls in blood sugar and energy levels. Yes, I included fats. Eating a meal totally devoid of fat can be less than satisfying. Fats provide satiation and staying power in your meal. Healthy oils in moderate amounts actually improve health and longevity. You can read more about this and obtain references in Chapters 12 and 18. Providing your body with balanced meals will increase satisfaction and decrease food cravings.

Variety

Variety is said to be the spice of life, but it works the other way around, too: spice can add variety to your life. Eating is not meant to provide just fuel to keep us going. It is also meant to be an enjoyable experience. And just as we need variety in other areas of life, we need it in the color, tastes, temperatures, and textures of the foods we eat, as well as in the types of foods themselves. Eating the same foods day after day becomes boring and uninteresting; it causes us to pay less attention to what and how we are eating and can actually be unhealthy.

One of the most frequent causes of food sensitivities is eating the same foods over and over. Bread, cereal, and pasta may sound like variety, but they aren't if they are all made out of wheat. Cereal and milk, creamed soup and lasagna may sound like variety, but they are not if they all contain dairy products. Seek out a wide variety of foods. Switch from beef to pork to chicken to emu. Try rye crackers and quinoa pasta and oatmeal. We have become very set in our ways and often feel too tired to change them. The fact is if we'd change them we probably wouldn't be so tired!

Of the six tastes listed in Chapter 10, we Americans include far more than we need of the sweet and salty tastes and very few of the others. Isn't it interesting that the four tastes we ignore—bitter, astringent, pungent, and sour—are found mostly in low-fat, high-fiber foods that stimulate the metabolism? Adding a variety and balance of tastes to your meals can facilitate better nutrition and loss of excess body fat.

It is also important to include a variety of natural colors, textures, and temperatures. Color provides eye appeal to your meals and can also increase the nutritional value. This is true because the bright colors found in food are from fresh vegetables and fruits that are nutrient dense. Food can be crunchy, liquid, thick and smooth, or chewy. I personally have experienced satisfaction with a meal but have still been driven to a food for its texture. My mouth, not my brain or my stomach, was driving me. I needed to crunch on something. A desperate need to crunch or chew or tear at food can be caused by not eating many crunchy foods, or more commonly by stress. Crunching, chewing, and tearing are very stress relieving. As you become more balanced in your life, this need will be reduced. A strong desire for smooth creamy foods or foods you can suck on can be an indication of a lack of these textures in your diet, or more likely it is a need to be soothed and comforted. These kinds of textures represent the comfort of infancy when everything was warm, smooth, creamy.

As you love yourself, and take better care of yourself in non-food ways, you will lose this drive. I used to be in the ranks of millions of Americans that use ice cream to soothe away pain. Five years ago I could and would eat a half gallon of ice cream in one sitting. Although I still keep ice cream in my freezer most of the time, I now handle my comfort needs on a regular basis, before they drive me to food. Nowadays a half gallon of ice cream dies of freezer burn before it is finished. Eating food to relieve stress or give comfort when you are not physically hungry leads to excess body fat. However, remember that eliminating comfort eating before you develop a new behavior pattern to handle your psychological needs leads to pain and frustration. Work on loving and comforting yourself and destressing your body, mind, and spirit first, and you will gradually lose the need to eat for comfort.

Finding that place in your eating experiences where you feel satisfied, balanced, and energized and then putting your fork down is one of the most important skills you can learn. You will eat past satisfaction often when you start actively paying attention. However, the fact that you notice that you are eating past satisfaction is progress toward health. Noticing, becoming aware of what you are doing, is the first step in the process of growth and change. Do not berate yourself or feel guilty for eating past satisfaction. If you do this, you will want to stop noticing because it is painful. Noticing, paying attention, and being aware are the keys to change. Applaud yourself for noticing.

Look at eating past satisfaction with curiosity. Take the preceding list and see what is missing from your meals. Take a look at your life. What might you be trying to fill or hide by overeating? Use your awareness for growth. We have found that our clients begin to identify when they are hungry fairly easily but that stopping when their physical needs are satisfied is more challenging, largely because they are not used to being fulfilled or satisfied in any area of life. Does this apply to you? You may be less than satisfied in your job, your relationships, your self-worth and attempting to make this up by overfilling yourself with food. Not because you are weak-willed but because your body-mind-spirit system is driven to find pleasure and happiness.

When pleasure and happiness are lacking in one area of life, we invariably seek it in another. For example, the person who has an unsatisfying marriage may become a workaholic. This drive to be pleasured and fulfilled is innate. When it feels as if our everyday life is not satisfying or pleasurable, we turn to artificial pleasures. Some people seek comfort, pleasure, or excitement through drugs, others through alcohol, sex, or gambling. Still others seek it through food. Whatever direction this misguided search takes, the answer to ending the search is inside ourselves. It involves recognizing and honoring our spirit, our inner self, the self that is loving and loved, the self that is willing, deserving, giving, and striving toward growth. There is not one drug, drink, food, or person that can fill our need to love and accept ourselves.

Opportunities for Growth

Awareness

- Notice what causes you to put down your fork and stop eating. Is it external cues like the time, a clean plate, dessert, or the fact that others are done? Is it internal cues, such as feeling full, satisfied, uncomfortable, that your belt is tight? If it is "fullness," notice when you stand up how full you are: 0, +1, +2, +5? Also notice if 10 minutes later you feel even fuller. Practice hunger and satisfaction awareness often.

- Check the clock when you start eating. How long are your meals? Compare sit-down meals with fast-food meals.

- Look at your meals. How do they rate in the elements that contribute to satisfaction? Are you really hungry when you start? Are you eating what you have an appetite for? Are you paying attention to your food? Are you eating quality food and pacing yourself? Do you have a variety of foods, colors, tastes, and textures?

Introspection

- Consider the possibility that there are very important areas of your life—job, family, relationships, time for yourself—that are unfulfilling right now and you may be trying to fill them with food. What small steps can you take to begin making these areas of your life more satisfying?

- Are there other unhealthy ways—alcohol, drugs, sex, smoking, gambling—that you try to pleasure yourself with besides food? Could these be artificial attempts to find satisfaction and pleasure in a life that is sorely lacking?

Old Beliefs to Let Go

- I can never be satisfied with small amounts of healthy foods.

- Eating between meals is bad.

- I don't have time for sit-down, knife-and-fork meals.

- Feeling satisfaction before I'm full is difficult.

- I feel bad when I overeat.

New Beliefs to Embrace

- I am perfectly satisfied with small amounts of healthy foods.

- I enjoy a wide variety of foods, spices, textures, and colors in my meals.

- I always have time to eat slowly and nourish my body.

- I look for a learning experience anytime I eat past my own sense of satisfaction.

- I easily feel the point of balance and satisfaction when I eat.

- I know when I'm satisfied, and I immediately end my eating experience.

Vividly Imagine

- Take the image of savoring that you created in the last chapter and add to it the sense of satisfaction, balance, energy, the knowing that it is time to put down your fork. Imagine when you do this that there is food left on the plate. Add a clock to your image and notice the time when you start eating. When you put your fork down, notice that 20 minutes have passed on the clock since you began your meal. Feel the lightness of satisfaction and compare it with the awful feeling of having overeaten. Release any fears of eating such small amounts and promise yourself you can have something to eat the very next time you are hungry, whether it is mealtime or not.

Patterns for Action

• Decrease the number of fast-food and hold-in-your-hand meals that you have per week and increase the number of sit-down, knife-and-fork 20- to 25-minute meals you eat.

• Have balanced, nutritious between-meal snacks and mini-meals available. Don't get caught having to use the vending machine if you can help it.

• Look at your food and make mental or physical lines in it at the size serving you think will satisfy you based on your hunger level. Eat to those lines and note your level of satisfaction. If you decide to eat the rest, note your level of satisfaction then. Note your level of fullness 20 minutes after the meal. Which point felt best?

Additional Reading

Meal Satisfaction
Chopra, Deepak, M.D. *Perfect Weight*. New York: Harmony Books, 1994.

Relationship Satisfaction
Lerner, Harriet G., Ph.D. *The Dance of Intimacy*. New York: Harper and Row, 1989.

Job Satisfaction
Sinetar, Marsha. *Do What You Love, the Money Will Follow*. New York: Dell, 1987.

Habit 9: Develop a Basic Understanding of Nutrition

We are all quite willing to learn the fuel and maintenance requirements of a new car. Why do we resist learning the fuel and maintenance requirements of our own bodies? If your car falls apart from neglect, it can be replaced. Your body can't.

THE WEIGHT OF an average American has been increasing every year for the last 10 years. This is not solely because we are eating more, but also because we are eating more poorly. The foods we eat are so bereft of nutrients that we keep eating more in an attempt to meet our nutritional needs. The problem is we eat more of the same poor-quality food, so we get fat instead of nourished. The only way to get out of this unhealthy cycle is to take responsibility for knowing the general nutritional value of the food we are eating. We do not need to memorize and count calories or fat grams. We just need to increase our awareness.

Learning about nutrition can strike fear in the hearts of the bravest among us. Even those with multiple college degrees cringe at the thought of reading a food label and actually *knowing* what it is they are eating. That's because most of us really don't want to know. If we knew, we might be so appalled that we would be forced to change what we eat! It's not the knowledge of nutrition that turns people off; it's the fear of changing their habits. Read this chapter with an open mind and read about the process of change later. We believe that anyone, with just a bit of desire, can develop a practical understanding of food and nutrition.

You Don't Have to Be a Health Nut to Be Healthy

What is nutrition anyway? The dictionary defines *nutrition* as the process of taking in and utilizing food for growth and development. In this chapter we will discuss the food we choose to take in, and in Chapter 18 we will look more closely at how this food is utilized. This chapter is about awareness. It is about looking at what you eat and deciding whether your food choices are growth producing or just girth producing. Among the naturally slim people we interviewed, some had an in-depth understanding of nutrition. However, most of them had only a very basic knowledge of nutrition and the majority were open to hearing new nutritional information that could be beneficial to their health. When these same naturally slim people read about nutrition, it was because they had a healthy love and respect for their bodies, not because they felt they had to. They read articles about nutrition with curiosity, and they did not jump on and off supplements and diets based on the latest magazine article. Knowledge about nutrition gives us the power to choose what we eat with intelligence.

Let's look at a popular nutrition topic: fat in the diet. A naturally slim person might read about which oils are essential to good health and which ones are harmful. She would get her information from several sources and then maybe talk to a nutritionist or a health care professional for validation. After that she would look at the fats she was eating and compare them with the list of healthy and unhealthy fats. Maybe she'd be surprised at how much unhealthy fat she was consuming and look at where she might make some changes. Then slowly she would start buying different products and trying them or begin ordering a little differently at restaurants. She would try her new habit on for size and work it into her life slowly. Gradually the change would be assimilated, leaving her with little conscious memory of having eaten differently in the past.

In contrast, many of our clients tend to read a single magazine article and then run out to buy the latest fat-burning supplement or liquid appetite suppressant. They jump right in with little knowledge or forethought, frequently because their self-esteem is low. They believe that the author of any published article must know more than they do. They seek external advice and feedback rather than trusting themselves to make an intelligent decision from within. People who do not love and respect themselves may give others the gifts of time and patience, but they rarely give these gifts to themselves. If you fit this description, please go back to Habit 2 on self-love. The impulsive approach you may have been taking to nutrition might work for a few people, but most of us succeed in making permanent change only through knowledge, validation, planning, and fully informed choice.

So, what constitutes a good basic knowledge of nutrition? According to *Infotrack Magazine Index,* in the years 1988 to 1995, 3,755 magazine articles on nutrition were published—not including medical and professional journals. Also in print were 1,133 articles on diets, 1,026 on weight loss, and 19,129 articles on food. Would you need to read all of these to acquire an everyday working knowledge of food and nutrition? Of course not. We feel very strongly that the nutritional information needed to begin to make healthy food choices can be kept pretty fundamental. Basically it's a simple matter of awareness—(1) knowing the origin of what you eat, (2) understanding how nutrient dense your usual diet is, and (3) getting a feel for the balance or imbalance in your food intake. In this chapter we will cover topics (1) and (2); topic (3) will be addressed in detail in Chapter 18. You are welcome to seek information about nutrition elsewhere. Indeed, as you change your beliefs about the subject of nutrition, you may develop a desire to know more about how your wonderful body works (see Additional Readings at the end of Chapter 18).

Overweight People Need Food, Too!

Overweight people and chronic dieters spend a lot of time focusing on what is wrong with their bodies. What about what is right with them? Our bodies are absolute miracles of dynamic equilibrium. We are constantly burning calories to keep us warm, digest our food, create new cells, and replace whole organs cell by cell over several years. Without a conscious thought we keep breathing, our hearts keep beating, and our muscle reflexes keep working. Our bodies, no matter what size, are absolute miracles. Anything you can learn about your body to help you appreciate this is much more beneficial than counting fat grams.

Start by understanding that all human beings are energy manifest. Absolutely every part of us down to the subatomic level is in motion at all times. We are building and tearing down at every level, from cells to organs; we are digesting and creating; we are formulating and secreting; we are dreaming, learning, feeling, and dancing—just to name a few of the energetic functions going on at any given time. Yet very often overweight people think of themselves as low-energy people. True, their metabolisms may be a little slower than others', but still they are truly energetic, and that condition requires them to eat.

I can remember as a yo-yo dieter feeling very righteous when I went all day without eating. After all, I reasoned, I had a slow metabolism. I didn't need much food and would rather be burning fat anyway. That reasoning was erroneous. *We all need to eat.* We can't burn fat unless we have the nutrients necessary to do it. Starving ourselves merely lowers our ability to burn calories—any kind of calories, fat or otherwise.

If we all need to eat, what should we eat? If you have been involved in dieting, you have come to rely on the dictates of other people. You have abdicated your personal power and your ability to interpret your own body signals to a book, a magazine, a doctor, or a program. You don't need that kind of help. What you may need, however, is knowledge about what foods are health building and nutrient dense and what foods are not health building and are nutrient challenged. Once you have this information in an easy-to-understand form you can compare what you are eating, meal by meal or day by day, with this information and make your own decisions about where you might want to eat differently.

Quality: Getting the Most Nutrition per Bite

Every piece of food, no matter what shape or size, usually has some sort of nutrient value, a nutrient being a substance that provides nourishment and enhances cell growth and development. Nutrients include both macronutrients (proteins, carbohydrates, and fat) and micronutrients (vitamins and minerals), and the level of these constituents in food determines its quality. Instead of looking at the quantity of food you are eating, begin to look at that quality. Nutrient-dense food gives you the most growth enhancement per bite. Diets that focus on quantity alone leave you very hungry and offer little chance of success because when food quality is low, you will naturally tend to increase the quantity you eat to try to make up for it. Therefore advice to take smaller portions will be effective only for someone who is already eating a nutrient-dense diet.

The nutritional quality of a food varies greatly depending on how the food is grown, stored, processed, and prepared for consumption. In this fast-paced society, cooking is often cast aside for convenience. We rely on processed, prepared, fast, and restaurant foods, with little thought about the quality of the fuel we put into our bodies. Fortunately you can rely on several general rules to give you a feel for whether your food is nutrient dense or nutrient challenged.

Whole Foods Versus Partial Foods

The more a food resembles its form when hanging on the tree, dangling from the bush, or rooting under the ground, the more life, energy, and nutrition it contains. Whole foods are those that have not been altered since they left their source. You can cut, chop, or pulverize a whole food, and no nutrients will be lost as long as it is consumed in a short period of time. However, when apples are made into apple pie or wheat is made into white bread, the life of the food and many of its nutrients are lost.

Nutrient loss occurs when parts of the whole food are removed and again when the food is cooked or processed. In the case of the apple, removing the skin removes vitamins and fiber; cooking the apple causes further nutrient loss. The greatest loss occurs with boiling. In the case of whole wheat processed into white flour, removing the hull removes fiber, and removing the germ removes vitamins, minerals, oils, and protein. What is left is the starchy white part of the grain that contains little nutritional value. The carbohydrates found in white flour are so refined that they can enter the bloodstream almost as fast as refined sugar. This causes huge shifts in blood sugar levels, leading to excess insulin secretion, sugar cravings, and storage of fat.

But whole foods are desirable also because we really don't know what else we may be missing when we divide them into parts. Scientists measure the vitamins, minerals, carbohydrates, fats, and proteins in foods to classify their nutritional value, but they still can't describe the role of some 350 phytochemicals found in whole fruits and vegetables. They still cannot artificially reproduce a carrot. Why? Because the whole of any living thing is greater than the sum of its parts. This goes for humans as well as vegetables. You are more than blood and bones and flesh, and an apple is more than carbohydrate, fiber, and vitamins. We may wait a very long time before science isolates the life force that runs through all of us living things. That is why whole people need whole foods: they have a life and an energy that cannot be measured or replaced by a tablet. Taking beta-carotene capsules will never provide the nourishment and cancer-fighting capabilities of a raw carrot.

Live Food Versus Dead Food

With the premise that a sense of humor can be as important as a sense of nutrition in the process of becoming slim, I give you this poem:

> *Ashes to ashes,*
> *Dust to dust,*
> *Dead food is for fertilizer,*
> *Not for us.*

A live food means just that. It is live, unaltered by storage or processing. It contains that immeasurable life force we mentioned in the previous paragraphs. You can plant an apple in the ground and an apple tree will grow from it. You can't do the same with applesauce! The same is true in the case of a raw peanut versus a roasted peanut, a raw zucchini versus zucchini bread, or raw whole-grain granola versus whole-grain bread. Each step of processing causes a loss of life and measurable nutrients. The fact that live foods are better for your health than dead foods does not mean you have to empty your freezer and become a truck farmer. Nor does it mean that you should skip this chapter because you have never eaten nor do you intend to eat a raw vegetable. Strive for moderation, movement forward, and balance. This is a process. Give up judgment and just read for information. If this book doesn't make you a little uncomfortable, then you probably aren't growing.

The following is a list of food-processing techniques in descending order of their ability to preserve the original nutritional value of a food:

Live, fresh, raw

⬇ Fresh frozen

⬇ Fresh dried

⬇ Quick cooked

⬇ ⬇ Quick cooked, then frozen

⇩ ⇩ ⇩ Fully cooked

⇩ ⇩ ⇩ ⇩ Fully cooked and frozen

⇩ ⇩ ⇩ ⇩ ⇩ Fully cooked and canned

Raw foods contain naturally occurring enzymes that our systems need to digest and utilize the nutrients to the fullest. When we cook a food, we kill the enzymes, putting a burden on our digestive system. Recently scientists observed that when cooked foods are eaten there is almost an allergic-type response that occurs in the body, with an accompanying increase in white blood cells. However, if a meal contains at least 20 percent raw food, that reaction does not occur—a good reason to eat a salad with your cooked meals. The nutritional value of cooked preserved food can be decreased even further by overcooking or crowding out nutrients with fat-laden sauces, chemicals, and preservatives. In contrast, the nutritional value of a fresh raw seed, bean, or grain can be increased tremendously by allowing it to sprout. The protein content in a sprouted seed or bean is increased by 15 to 30 percent, along with an increase in chlorophyll, fiber, vitamin C, niacin, riboflavin, all the B vitamins, and beta-carotene.

We are not suggesting that all your meals should be live raw foods. *Always* and *never*, along with perfection and obsession, have no place in the process of becoming healthy and slim. However, adding a salad or some other raw vegetable to your cooked meals and a piece of raw fruit to your whole-grain cereal might be a healthy measure to consider. Those of you who have dieted may need some extra time to assimilate raw foods because they were pushed so very hard on every diet you were on. After I quit dieting it took me a very long time to enjoy a carrot stick or a piece of fresh fruit. Many of us overused raw foods because they were on the "unlimited list" of every diet we ever went on. It may take a while to change those diet perceptions.

Naked Food Versus Dressed Food

The actual nutritional value of a food, cooked or raw, does not change by adding sauces, gravies, dips, or dressings. However, many sauces and gravies are made of mostly oil or fat. If you have prepared a balanced meal, the additional fat may cause your hunger to be satisfied before you finish the other nutrient-dense foods on your plate. Except for certain essential fats found in small amounts of high-quality fish and vegetable oils, fat serves as a storage unit for excess calories to be used in the future. Sauces and gravies add variety and taste to foods but little nutritional value.

If you dress your food, dress it lightly and sparingly. You have already cooked your food to death—no need to smother it, too! There are some wonderful light, broth-based sauces containing appealing tidbits like capers and olives and raisins that can dress up a food with minimal fat. Play with your food, have fun, and don't be a martyr. If you believe that you can't live without gravy on your potatoes, work on some other health change. There is always something you can do.

Lean Food Versus Fat Food

Most Americans, including the authors, eat meat. If you have chosen to be a vegetarian, that is fine. If you are a vegetarian but you feel deprived every time a friend has a hamburger or you dream about eating fried chicken, you may want to evaluate both your motives and your nutrition. Being a vegetarian does not mean you can't gain weight. Cheeses, nuts, seeds, dairy products, and potato chips can all be considered "vegetarian," and all contain a large amount of fat. Being a vegetarian requires an increased knowledge of nutrition to ensure that you get an adequate intake of iron and protein.

One of the worst things you can do is to look at fat alone when changing the way you eat. Fat does not exist alone. Often when people cut out fat, they stop eating meat without learning how to get adequate protein from grains and legumes. Beef, fish, chicken, and turkey are very concentrated sources of protein. Protein is an important nutrient we often forget about in the current high-carbohydrate, low-fat eating craze.

If you do eat meat, begin to choose lean over fat. Fat in meat is relatively hidden so that we aren't as aware of it as we would be if we were adding butter or oil to it. Lean beef is available and can be very tasty. In fowl, dark meat has more fat than light, but if you love dark meat, pay more attention to the amount you are eating. It is the amount as well as the type of meat you eat that can contribute to excess body fat.

It's also important not to lump together all fats and oils. Plant sources of oil are much healthier than animal sources. Olive oil and canola oil are healthier than butter, cream, and fatty meat. If you love butter, look at the amounts and where the taste of butter matters, then replace it in areas you can live with. Certain fish oils are extremely beneficial to health.

No-fat and *low-fat* are the buzzwords of the decade, and it all makes sense: to lose fat, eat less fat; to lose more fat, eat even less fat. It is true that we Americans have generally eaten much more fat than we need, but we do need some fat. Viewing fat as bad in any form causes problems of its own. You may not know this, but there are many people out there getting fat on low-fat diets! When you buy no-fat cakes, cookies, ice cream, and crackers, you don't fool yourself for very long. The nutrition in these foods is very poor (the taste can be even worse). They are usually made of highly processed white flour, sugar or artificial sweeteners, and a very long list of chemicals added to try to make them palatable. They are some of the deadest foods I have ever met! These foods are usually very poor imitations of the real thing and provide so little satisfaction that people will eat two or three times as much as they normally would.

Even if you have no fat in your diet, you can still gain weight if you are eating more calories than you are burning up. As great as this no-fat ruse may seem, you cannot eat unlimited amounts of dead carbohydrates and lose weight. Unlimited amounts of vegetables, yes. Unlimited amounts of no-fat chips, bagels, and cookies, no.

Organically Raised Food Versus Conventionally Raised Food

It is a fact that the state of the soil or water a food grows in will directly affect its nutritional value. This makes sense. If a potato is grown in mineral-depleted soil, it will not have the same amount of minerals as a potato grown in mineral-rich soil. Most of our farmlands have been overplanted and repeatedly covered with fertilizers and insecticides. Food grown conventionally can never be as safe and healthy as food that is grown organically, partly because of fertilizers and insecticides that remain in the soil for years and partly because we do not know the long-term effects of the chemicals used now. This food of questionable safety, along with huge amounts of hormones and antibiotics, is also fed to the animals that give us eggs, milk, and meat, leaving those products of questionable safety as well. Organic farmers are dedicated to providing the highest-quality food using methods that protect both human health and the health of the environment. They use natural fertilizers, renewable resources, and recycled materials and are dedicated to replenishing and maintaining long-term soil fertility.

Documented differences in mineral content of organic versus conventionally grown produce are astounding. Organically grown snap beans, cabbage, lettuce, and tomatoes contain three to five times as much calcium, magnesium, potassium, and manganese as do their conventionally grown counterparts. These same organically grown vegetables contain 20 to 40 times as much copper and 20 to 40 times as much iron!

Many of you may never have set foot in a "health food" store and may consider the extra expense of organic food to be prohibitive. Suppose you figured the cost of your food based on its nutritional quality? Suppose an organic orange gave you 50 percent more nutrients for only a 10 percent increase in cost. Wouldn't it be worth it? "But the organic stuff never looks as good as the other," you may say. That's because certified organic farms do not use chemical pesticides or put coloring into orange skins. They are concerned with quality over eye appeal. You may have wondered why your grocer's beautiful red tomatoes taste like cardboard. Try an organic tomato and see if you can taste the difference.

Are Your Meals Nutrient Dense or Nutrient Challenged?

We have developed a simple system to help you get a general picture of the nutrient density of your food intake. Have fun with the Nutrient Density Evaluation Chart on pages 148–49, play with it, and use it for information, not judgment or guilt. You can use it to plot a meal, a day of meals, or even a whole week's worth. Just follow these directions:

1. After you eat, count how many servings you had of vegetables, fruits, grains, legumes, nuts, meats, dairy, and eggs. One serving is approximately:

> Vegetables—1 cup raw, 2/3 cup cooked
>
> Fruit—1 medium piece raw, 1/2 cup cooked
>
> Grains—1 slice white/light bread; 1/2 piece heavy bread, bagel, muffin, croissant; 1/2 cup cooked grains, potatoes, legumes (beans, peas, lentils), or corn
>
> Nuts and seeds—2 tablespoons whole, 1 tablespoon butter
>
> Dairy and eggs—1 cup non-fat or 1/2 cup other, 1 ounce cheese, 1 egg
>
> Meat, fish, poultry—3 to 4 ounces (the size of a deck of playing cards)
>
> Sweeteners, fats, and oils—1 teaspoon

We know that in the real world people really don't want to weigh or measure their food, which is why you fill this chart in after you eat and should only approximate amounts. If you have no idea what a serving is, sometime when you are in the kitchen just play with teaspoons, tablespoons, cups, and ounces. Start to get a feel for various serving sizes. Begin to notice the amounts that you put on your plate and eat. A 16-ounce steak is not one serving of meat, but four servings.

2. Place an X in the Nutrient Density Evaluation Chart for each serving of each food, under the nutrient density category that most accurately reflects how your serving was processed or prepared. For example: A whole apple eaten raw with the skin on gets an X under fruits in the "whole" category. A croissant gets an X under grains in the category labeled "white flour, baked with fat added," all the way on the right. If you don't know what the food you are eating is made of, there are three things you can do: (1) Ask the person who prepared it. (2) Read the ingredient label on the package. (3) Buy a book that lists the nutrient contents of foods. If you are reading ingredient labels, note that the ingredients are listed in descending order of content in that food. (If enriched flour is listed first and whole-wheat flour is fourth, the food should be plotted under white flour, because that is its major ingredient.)

3. When you're finished plotting your meals, look at the pattern of your food choices. Where are most of your food choices located? Do you eat a lot of nutrient-dense foods? Do you eat more nutrient-challenged foods? Feel free to make several photocopies of this blank chart for your personal use.

Hopefully this chart will give you an easy, pleasurable way to view your current nutritional intake. Look at your meals and see if there is a place where you might begin to increase the nutrient density of your food. With this system, instead of taking away foods, you are adding nutrients. It is a much more positive way to look at food. Food keeps you alive! It is not an enemy to be eliminated. It is a gift to your body from yourself. Your body, regardless of shape or size, deserves food of the highest quality.

NUTRIENT DENSITY EVALUATION CHART

Nutrient Dense				Nutrient Challenged
VEGETABLES				
Whole, Fresh, Raw	Fresh, Lightly Cooked	Frozen, Lightly Cooked	Cooked Soft, Canned	Cooked with Fats or Sugars
FRUITS				
Whole, Fresh, Raw	Fresh, Lightly Cooked	Frozen, Lightly Cooked	Cooked Soft, Canned	Cooked with Fats or Sugars
GRAINS				
Whole, Unprocessed	Whole, Flaked, Cooked	Mixed Whole and Refined Breads and Pastas	Fully Refined Breads and Pastas	Fully Refined, Added Fats and Sugars
NUTS, SEEDS, AND LEGUMES				
Raw, Sprouted	Whole, Raw	Gently Cooked or Dry Roasted	Roasted in Oil	Roasted or Cooked with Added Fats, Salt, Sugars

Eggs

Cooked with Little or No Fat	—	Cooked with Butter	—	Cooked with Butter, Cheese, and Meat

Dairy Products

Skim, Nonfat	1%, 2%, Low-Fat	Part-Skim Cheese	Whole-Milk Cheese	Ice Cream, Butter, Cream, Sugar Added

Meat, Fish, and Fowl

Lean Fish, White Meat	95% Lean Beef or Pork, Dark Meat	85% Lean Beef, Fatty Fish	75% Lean Hamburger, Pork Ribs, Steak	Meats with Visible Fat, Fried, with Gravy

Fats and Oils

Monounsaturated, Vegetable Oils	—	Polyunsaturated, Vegetable Oils	—	Saturated Fats and Hydrogenated Oils

Sweeteners

Cooked Pureed Whole Fruit	—	Honey, Dried Cane Syrup, Molasses	White Sugar, Corn Syrup	Chemical Sweeteners

Opportunities for Growth

Awareness

- This whole chapter is about awareness. Photocopy the preceding chart and begin plotting some of your meals. Become aware of the nutrient density of your meals.

- Begin reading food labels for nutrients and balance.

Introspection

- What are your feelings about nutrition?

- If your beliefs are less than positive, are you willing to consider changing them?

- Is there one small step you are willing to take to increase the nutritional density of your eating?

Old Beliefs to Let Go

- Nutrition is complicated and hard to learn.

- We're all going to die sometime, so I'm going to eat whatever I want and enjoy it.

- It's good if I don't eat anything.

- I need someone to tell me what I should and shouldn't eat.

- I hate raw foods, especially vegetables.

New Beliefs to Embrace

- It's easy to identify and choose nutrient-dense foods.

- I want to live.

- I enjoy choosing and eating nutritious foods.

- I naturally desire raw fruits and vegetables.

- Learning about my body's nutritional needs brings me great joy.

- I enjoy frequently shopping for fresh food.

Vividly Imagine

- Imagine yourself getting in the car and driving to the food store. Be sure you're smiling. Shopping for fresh food for yourself is fun. Go into the store, take a cart, and steer away from the canned and processed foods. Start selecting vegetables and fruits. Pick each one up, look at it, and smell it. Imagine how you will cook it. Then go and select some fresh chicken and fish. Savor the experience of shopping.

- Review the visual images that you created in the savoring and satisfaction habits (Chapters 7 and 8). Be sure that the plate of food you are eating in these images is filled with nutrient-dense foods. Two different vegetables, a serving of meat, and a serving of grain is one example of a balanced meal (Chapter 18 covers balanced nutrition in more detail). Remove the sauces and decrease the butter in your image and make healthy substitutes. Feel satisfied without as much fat.

Patterns for Action

- When you are trying to decide what to eat, ask yourself, "Have I had anything fresh or live to eat today?"

- After you've plotted some of your meals and have a good feel for where your nutrition is challenged, commit to moving at least one food group one step to the left. Take one small step toward improving your nutrition. Create this habit before you tackle another food group or another step to the left.

- Visit a health food store. Start to put that store into your image.

- Begin to keep fresh fruit and vegetables in your house. If they go bad before you eat them, throw them out and buy some more. Have them available.

Additional Reading

Townsley, Cheryl. *Food Smart.* Pinon Press, 1994.
Wittenberg, Margaret. *Good Food: The Complete Guide to Eating Well.* Freedom, CA: The Crossing Press, 1995.

See Chapter 18 for more readings on nutrition.

THIRTEEN

Habit 10: Play Every Day

*When nutritious food feels satisfying and
exercise feels like play, there will be no soldiers
left in the battle of the bulge.*

NATURALLY SLIM PEOPLE, like children, enjoy moving their bodies. They are aware of their bodies' natural desire to alternate periods of rest with periods of activity. If they have been sitting too long and feel stiff, they get up, stretch, and walk around. If they have a job where they are not physically active, they try to get in sports, walking, or some other sort of play several times a week. They do this because it makes them feel good, not to keep themselves slim. Very few of the people we interviewed belonged to health clubs, and none of them had personal trainers. Usually they were involved in some sort of active exercise three to five days a week, but they were not compulsive about it. When naturally slim people who enjoyed daily walks were asked what they did about their exercise routines if they were sick or it was pouring rain, they laughed and said they didn't go.

Moving Your Body Is Natural and Enjoyable

As in many other areas of our lives, we have dozens of thoughts and beliefs about exercise that keep us from doing what we have a natural tendency to do:

Exercise is hard work.

Exercise is boring and tedious.

Exercise takes too much time.

Exercise is painful.

I'm too fat to exercise.

If I don't exercise every day, it won't do me any good.

If I don't do it fast enough, hard enough, or often enough to burn fat or improve my cardiovascular fitness, I might as well not do it.

If it's not at a gym or with an instructor, or at least done with a videotape, it's not really exercise.

If I don't sweat profusely and get short of breath and/or feel pain, I haven't had a real workout.

Moving your body is part of your nature. Our ancestors worked hard and ate heartily, and obesity was not an issue. Now we eat heartily and sit. We have not adapted our eating patterns to our lifestyle or our lifestyle to our eating patterns. We were not born to sit 16 hours a day. We have strong, capable muscles that thrive on activity and wither with disuse. Moving your body can be enjoyable, fun, and invigorating even though you may not believe it right now. Think of those naturally slim three- and four-year-olds who dance in front of the stereo for the sheer joy of it or run to a friend's house instead of walking just because they feel like it. Those three- and four-year-olds are you! There is nothing stopping you from enjoying physical activity just as much as they do. Nothing, that is, except the state of your mind. It is all of your negative beliefs about exercise that keep you from starting. It is all of your judgmental thoughts about not being good enough that keep you from continuing, and it is all your feelings of guilt that keep you from starting again after you've stopped. Your spirit and body are willing, but your state of mind won't let you.

Understand that your personal exercise program is yours and nobody else's. You can choose to play wherever and whenever you like and for as long as you like based on what you can do and feel good about. Your program may be to take a 10-minute walk three times a week. If that is more than you are doing now, then you are moving in the direction of health. Walk for those 10 minutes and enjoy every step. If you spend the 10-minute walk feeling guilty because you are not doing more, or looking at the marathon runners going by and thinking, What's the use? you are unlikely to keep up that exercise. If you stay focused on enjoying the walk and how good it makes you feel, you are much more likely to continue the activity on some sort of regular basis.

The great thing about exercise is that if you get started, at a level where you enjoy it and feel successful, you are very likely to *want* to stick with it. It makes perfect sense: if it's pleasurable, you'll be attracted to it; if it's painful, you won't be. Later you may enjoy it to the point that you are willing to push on that comfort zone and go for some growth, but starting out pushing your comfort zone may be the beginning of the end. As Deepak Chopra says in *Perfect Weight*, "Exercise should *produce* strength, energy and vitality, not use them up."

Preparing Your Mind

Before you take your first step on that first walk, support yourself with some new thinking. If you identify greatly with the beliefs listed earlier, choose some new ones like the ones at the end of this chapter. Next, choose an activity that you can imagine yourself doing for many years—an activity that can easily fit into your life, an activity you can imagine yourself enjoying.

Do some mental imaging about how you will look, feel, smell, and sound as you do this activity with pleasure and grace and a smile on your face. Remember, it's child's play; don't take it so seriously. Those of you who are not quite ready to be freewheeling may find a regular routine more comforting. If this is the case for you, then set up a regular routine. Make the routine realistic, even easy, to begin with to ensure a good feeling and learn to be OK if you have to break the routine. Being OK means guilt-free, judgment-free, and worry-free.

Preparing Your Body

Preparing your body for exercise can enhance the health benefits and the pleasurable feelings that you get from your session, whether it is 10 minutes or 60 minutes. Eating a balanced snack of some sort if you haven't eaten for a while is a good idea. Exercise can speed up your metabolism only if you are getting enough nutrition to support the extra energy requirements. If you have just had a meal, waiting 30 minutes before you exercise is sufficient. Stretching increases the blood flow to muscles and organs and helps prevent injury. Stretching is wonderful for you even if you haven't started exercising yet. Do a good overall body stretch like the Sun Salute found in *Perfect Weight* by Deepak Chopra or *Body, Mind and Sport* by John Douillard. Then do some specific stretches for the muscles and ligaments you will be using during each particular play session.

Take three big deep breaths, relax, take your first step, and enjoy. For those of you who have resisted exercise in the past because you overexerted and got short of breath, or for those who cannot walk up half of a flight of stairs or a mild incline without huffing and puffing, I have great news. I started out exactly like you, and the most powerful thing that ever happened to me was learning how to breathe when I exert myself. The process you need to learn is deep diaphragmatic breathing through your nose and a simple but noisy technique John Douillard calls "Darth Vader Breathing." After a little breathing practice I found that the mild inclines and stairs that I dreaded became a piece of cake!

I got to the top often breathing at the same rate as the one I had started at. Read *Body, Mind and Sport* to help dispel those old thoughts about exercise being breathless and painful.

Another trick I learned when walking stairs or inclines is to look at your feet or just ahead of them. When you focus on each step, the ground seems flat, or it seems like just one stair and thus isn't threatening. If you focus on the top of the stairs or the top of the hill ahead of you, a flood of *too hard, I can't,* and recollections of previous climbs that have left you breathless take over your mind and your body. You tighten up, feel stressed, breathe shallowly, and feel like quitting. Focus on each step and breathe deeply through your nose—a good philosophy for exercise and for life in general.

If you are eating well and have the willingness to exercise but feel you just don't have the energy, Brian Russell, a fitness consultant in Denver, recommends that you try taking a coenzyme supplement called Coenzyme Q_{10} (CoQ_{10}) or Ubiquinone CoQ_{10}. CoQ_{10} is an enzyme manufactured in the body and obtained from certain foods. This enzyme supports the bioenergetic functions in every single cell and is especially important to the energy factories in each cell called *mitochondria*. Studies have shown that the amount of CoQ_{10} we have available to our cells decreases with age and that low levels of CoQ_{10} can affect energy functions throughout the entire body.

When You Exercise, Be with Yourself

Whether you are lifting weights or taking a stroll, be with yourself in body, mind, and spirit. Pay attention to your body—it's the only way you can ever know whether what you are doing is producing stress or pleasure. Notice which muscles you are using and which you are not. If you are using only your legs, maybe you can figure out how to give your arms equal time. Notice any aches or pains; notice your breathing rate and heart rate. Even if you don't count them, you know what is comfortable. Exercising at a breath rate that allows you to talk while exercising is a good general indicator. Also, your heart should not be pounding in your ears at rates above 60 to 70 percent of maximum (maximum being 220 beats per minute minus your age). Darth Vader Breathing will improve your ability to take in more oxygen and get more of that oxygen to your heart.

If you like to listen to music when you exercise, do it to enhance your exercise, not to distract you from what you are doing. Also, exercising in beautiful surroundings, outdoors or with large windows and fresh air, increases the physical, mental, and spiritual nourishment you get from your session. Notice what is going on in your head. Is it quiet and totally involved in the experience? Or is it filled with thoughts about how hard this is, a project at work, the refrigerator's need for cleaning, or whether you will be done in time to beat rush hour traffic? When your head is filled with these thoughts, you experience the tension and stress of the thoughts instead of the invigorating effects of the exercise you are doing. When you used to think of exercise as painful, distracting your-self was a coping mechanism you used to avoid the pain. Now you don't need that coping mechanism, and in fact those thoughts take away from the positive benefits of your exercise.

Exercise and Fat Burning

We are willing to give you information about exercise and fat burning *only* if you promise to remember that this information does not necessarily make up some universal exercise plan that every overweight person *should* follow. We believe in being informed about health so as to make intelligent decisions. We do not believe in *always*, *every*, or *should*. You need to choose the way you want to exercise and how it will work the best for you so that it becomes a regular, pleasurable part of your life. Doing certain exercises just because they burn fat will not carry you through the years to come.

Personally, I get bored doing the same thing for exercise every day, though my mainstay is walking outdoors as often as I can. I add some dancing to CDs with my son, jumping on a small trampoline we have, and lifting weights once or twice a week. I find all of these enjoyable. However, I didn't start out that way. I started walking every day two years ago because I felt I *should*, and I quit because my life was too erratic for regular exercise. A year later I did a lot of belief change work using psychological kinesiology visualizations and affirmations about how "I love to move my body," "Exercise is easy and fun," and "Every time I move I increase my health and well-being." Gradually, without even consciously thinking about it, I found myself back outside, walking several times a week.

I picked up the book *Body, Mind and Sport*, became interested in the theories, and tried them out. Much to my amazement, once I learned how to breathe, I started climbing stairs occasionally—not to lose fat, but because I could! Months later I met Brian Russell, who taught me about strength and resistance training and how it assists in burning fat and preventing aging by causing growth hormone to be released. I agreed to try his new invention for resistance training called the Sand Dune and was amazed at the firmness my muscles achieved in only two weeks. At this time I started playing around with hand weights and dancing in my recreation room, too.

I did all this just for fun. Some weeks I do all of these different exercises; some weeks I do a few of them. When I was sick last winter, I didn't do anything except take an occasional walk for four weeks. But I always knew I'd get back to it, because I enjoy it, not because I should. Once you change that subconscious mind-set that has been repelling all forms of physical activity, you will begin attracting the information and the time and the inclination to exercise and play as often as you can.

As average Americans, we do ourselves a grave disservice when we think the only way to get any benefit from exercise is to train relentlessly, like athletes. For most people that will never be part of their life, but activity and play can be.

Our Ancestors Had the Right Idea

Have you ever noticed when watching movies about the Old West that there are no health clubs on Main Street, there are no cowboys or farmers running up and down the street in little silk shorts, and the saloon doesn't even serve light beer? What is the deal? Hadn't they ever heard of obesity? Our ancestors had to perform strength training and aerobic activity daily, and often for extended periods of time. "Lift that bale [strength training] and tote that barge [strength training and aerobic exercise]" were a way of life. They died young because of accidents and infections, not from diseases caused by poor diet and lack of activity.

We modern Americans need to pay attention to our activity level because our lifestyles rarely include lifting boulders, raking gardens, and washing clothes on a scrub board. Does that mean these times of convenience are "bad" and the old days were "good"? Of course not. The 20th century with all of its high-tech gadgets is a real kick! I, for one, am not about to give up my washing machine. We just need to tune away from the gadgets for a little while and tune in to ourselves. Moving our bodies, along with a balanced, nutrient-dense diet, can keep us physically young and functioning at top levels right up to the day we check out of here. You don't have to exercise to become an athlete. *Exercise for your health.*

Strength/Resistance Training

The word *train* means "to cause to grow as desired." We are daily training our body, causing it to grow as we desire. For years, whether we knew it or not, for some subconscious or unconscious reason, we desired to be overweight and we trained our body to do that. Now we desire it to grow in a different direction, away from fat and toward slim. So we must retrain it in the way it eats as well as the way it moves. In strength training we specifically want to cause our body to grow in the direction of strength, and the method we use is resistance. In life, when we meet a resistance we gather ourselves together, figure out how to overcome the resistance, and grow in strength in the process. Muscles work the same way. When a muscle meets a resistant force, it must gather all its resources together and overcome the resistance, and in the process it grows in strength. The greater the resistance, the greater the growth, in life and in muscles. The stronger we are, the more able we are to overcome the next resistance.

Strength training involves pitting your muscles against a resistant force on a regular basis and gradually increasing that force as the muscle adapts. You can use weights, circuit machines, elastic bands, a Sand Dune, or your own weight and gravity. Your muscles increase in strength by developing new muscle fiber. They will increase in tone and size with the increase in tissue and blood flow. Men's muscle development is greatly enhanced by the presence of the male hormone testosterone. Women will not get bulky like men with strength training.

Strength training can enhance overall health in anyone. It can be of particular help to chronic dieters because they often have lost a significant amount of muscle mass during their various states of dieting and starvation. Proper nutrition will ensure fat loss instead of muscle loss, and strength training can help you get back the firm, powerful, metabolically active muscle tissue you have lost through dieting and disuse. An increase of one pound of muscle can allow you to burn 50 to 100 more calories a day, even when you are sitting still. We begin to lose muscle mass at around 20 years of age, and unless we do some sort of exercising we can lose up to 5 percent of our muscle mass per year. If you are a chronic dieter or are middle-aged and haven't exercised in a long time, you may want to begin strength training to replace the muscle mass you have lost.

Strength training can also stimulate the release of growth hormone from the pituitary gland. Growth hormone stimulates tissue growth, metabolism, and a better fat-to-lean-muscle ratio. The best strength training works all major muscle groups in the body. If you are doing a limited amount of strength training, focus on the large locomotor muscles of the thigh. Training can be accomplished by lifting a weight, using a stretch band, or pushing down on the Sand Dune as many times as it takes to feel a particular muscle group getting tired and uncomfortable. For growth hormone release, push that muscle group a few more repetitions until you can feel a burning sensation for a minute or less. Then stop. A second and third set of these repetitions should be done to the same point of mild burn. You can also do the same type of exercise without any equipment, using your own weight and gravity as the resistance.

Stand straight with your knees comfortably apart. While keeping your shins straight up and down, drop your rear end down as if you were going to sit in a chair. In order to do this your torso will bend forward but your knees should stay aligned directly above your feet. In the beginning, squat to a point comfortable for balance and hold it until you feel your muscles start to quiver. Then stand up and squat again. Follow the same instructions concerning repetitions as described in the preceding paragraph. The effect of this exercise can be increased slowly over time by doing any or all of the following: deepening the squat position, increasing the time you hold the position, increasing the number of repetitions, or doing the squat with weights.

When you feel discomfort and push ahead into that burning sensation, your muscle will be forced to grow. Just as in life, when a situation makes us feel uncomfortable, it is an opportunity to grow. We can choose to stop and bypass the opportunity, or we can push through the discomfort we feel and force ourselves to grow. Neither way is right or wrong. If you stop the exercise before you experience the discomfort or the burning, you have still done something of benefit to your body. It is up to you to choose when and where you want to grow. Strength training may or may not be it.

Regular strength training stops muscle loss due to aging, decreases the incidence of osteoporosis and fractures, and indirectly increases our ability to burn fat. If you begin a regular program of strength training, you will need to increase your protein intake to assist your body's efforts to build new muscle tissue.

Aerobic Activity

Aerobic activity is the only activity that burns fat directly. *Aerobic* means "with oxygen," and fat can be burned only in the presence of oxygen. The activity can be walking, jogging, dancing, swimming, biking, chasing a child, carrying the laundry upstairs, and so on. During the first 20 minutes of exercise the body uses up glucose stored in the muscles. After that, fat is released from the cells as fatty acids and is used for energy. In the past people thought that the more out of breath you were during your exercise session, the better it was for you. This is not true if you are talking specifically about burning fat. Exercise periods that are 30 minutes or longer, with your heart rate at 60 to 70 percent of its maximum capacity, are the best fat burners.

Exercise Is the Fountain of Youth

Regular aerobic exercise can also decrease immobility and pain due to arthritis, decrease cholesterol, help normalize blood sugar levels, decrease incidence and symptoms of depression, decrease blood pressure, and improve PMS symptoms. It can increase your metabolism for hours afterward, and when coupled with strength training it can double your ability to burn fat. With all these wonderful benefits, why are 85 percent of Americans sedentary? Some are sedentary because they truly don't know how unhealthy it is to be sedentary. But most people are sedentary because of all the various thoughts and beliefs we listed in the beginning of this chapter. They perceive exercise as hard and cannot even imagine themselves doing it on a regular basis. Often they have jumped into exercise too vigorously in the past and burned themselves out, or they have friends who are exercise junkies and they don't want to live that way. The most unhealthy exercisers are those who exercise huge so that they can continue to eat huge. Remember, moderation and balance in all things. Regular exercise is invigorating and enjoyable; irregular exercise can be, too.

When you are ready to activate your natural desire to exercise, remember the following:

1. Change your belief system so that you begin to see exercise as positive.

2. Choose one activity or more that you feel you can enjoy now and for years to come. Begin to imagine yourself participating in that activity; imagine how you look, how you feel, and what you hear.

3. Choose the time and place you want to begin and make a date with yourself to play. If you miss the date, don't fret; just make another one.

4. Start at a level of exercise where you are sure you can experience pleasure and success.

5. Enjoy your moments of exercise, keeping the *shoulds* and *if onlys* out of your head.

6. After you are in a comfortable routine, check in with yourself periodically and see if you're ready to challenge that comfort zone and grow by adding some new dimension to your exercise.

You were born to move. Running, jumping, dancing, digging, raking, shoveling, and walking are part of your nature. We invite you to become reacquainted with the part of yourself that has always been active and fit, the part of you that is moving your body as play.

Opportunities for Growth

Awareness

- How often do you move your body during the day? Before work? After work? Would your job or lifestyle measure low or high if you were wearing a pedometer?

- Do you do specific things to avoid moving your body, like

parking as close as you can to the store, even in good weather?

- Is there any activity that you do just on the weekends or occasionally that you'd enjoy doing more of if you had the time? Gardening? Sports? Walking?

- When was the last time you did regular exercise? Why did you stop? Pain? Guilt? Money? You were expecting a particular result, like weight loss, and you didn't get it?

- When you think of exercising, do you get feelings of pleasure or feelings of pain? If it's feelings of pain, start changing your thoughts and beliefs.

Introspection

- What are your feelings about exercise? Write them down. Are they based on some sort of negative experience you had in the past such as high school gym? Sports? Aerobics class?

- What word can you use to describe exercise that will give you a pleasurable response? *Play? Dance? Move?*

Old Beliefs to Let Go

- Exercise is hard work and painful.

- Exercise is boring.

- If I don't exercise every day, I might as well not do it at all.

- I'm too fat to exercise.

- Walking doesn't really count as exercise.

- No pain, no gain.

New Beliefs to Embrace

You can substitute any sport or walking or whatever form of activity you choose for the word *exercise* in these belief statements.

- It is my nature to move my body, and I love doing it.

- Every time I move, walk, exercise, I increase my health and well-being.

- Exercise is easy and fun.

- I'm ready, willing, and able to make exercise a regular part of my life now.

- I have all the time I need to exercise.

Vividly Imagine

- Pick one form of moving your body you think you could enjoy on a fairly regular basis, such as walking, and build your visualization around that particular exercise. Choose the time of day you think you would like to do the activity and put that in the visualization also. Imagine yourself getting up in the morning (or whatever time you have chosen) and getting dressed, putting on your walking shoes, jacket, etc. See yourself in the real setting where you will be going to do the exercise. Take yourself along the trail, walking briskly. Feel the breeze, smell the fresh air, and feel your muscles tightening and your breath deepening. Make sure the feelings are pleasurable. When you're done, take yourself in for a hot shower and a massage if you like!

Patterns for Action

- Park farther away from the store when you go and pat yourself on the back for remembering to exercise.

- Take the time to think about an activity you would enjoy doing on a regular basis. Read a book about it (yes, there are books on walking). Buy the shoes, scout out the best places to do the activity, and set a start date for yourself. Make it play time, time for yourself and your health.

- If walking up more than four stairs or walking up a slight incline brings dread and breathlessness to mind, take the time to learn how to breathe. Even if it doesn't cause dread, take the time to learn how to breathe (read *Body, Mind and Sport*).

Additional Reading

Chopra, Deepak, M.D. *Perfect Weight*. New York: Harmony Books, 1994.

Diamond, Harvey, and Marilyn Diamond. *Fit for Life II*. New York: Warner Books, 1987.

Douillard, John. *Body, Mind and Sport*. New York: Crown, 1994.

Landis, Robyn. *Body Fueling*. New York: Warner Books, 1994.

FOURTEEN

A Habit Begins with a Thought

*Focusing on the breaking of old habits gives
them far more attention than they deserve.
The only way to get rid of an old habit is to
carefully construct a new one and never give
the old one another thought!*

NOW YOU HAVE IT: The 10 habits of naturally slim people, 10 habits to incorporate into your life that will make you slim forever. Easy as pie.

I don't know about you, but I never found making a pie easy. Maybe that old saying was referring to eating the pie—*that* I can identify with . . . "easy as *eating* a slice of pie." Wouldn't it be wonderful if we could bake these 10 habits into a pie and just by eating the pie make the 10 habits part of our lives? You've heard of humble pie? Well, this would be habit pie, and one pie would be sold with every self-help book.

Why are there are so many self-help books on the topic of losing weight? First, no single answer is right for every person. Second, there is no such thing as habit pie. People read book after book on the same subject, hoping that one of them will actually assist them in doing something differently. There is a lot of good information out there about different types of food and exercise for different types of people. However, there is very little guidance about how to make the information a part of your life. Often authors come across with the attitude "I've given you the answer; now just buckle down and do it!" Insight and knowing "how to" do not necessarily equate with change.

We vow not to leave you in that lurch. We have been there too many times ourselves. That is why the second half of this book is so important. Unless you understand how your current habits were formed and what is necessary to assimilate new habits into your life, *The Ten Habits of Naturally Slim People* will be one more "Oh, that's really interesting" self-help book to store on a shelf. We want you to use this book as an ongoing guide to changing your life in ways that will lead you to three-dimensional health in spirit, mind, and body. For years you have continued to do the same thing over and over, diet after diet, expecting the outcome to be different. Hopefully you are now ready to be aware of what you are thinking and doing so that you can, in fact, do something different.

What Is a Habit?

The dictionary defines a habit as "a regular, predictable, automatic pattern of action that has been acquired by frequent repetition." The key words are *action, acquired, repetition,* and *automatic.* A habit is an *action* or way of doing things that we were not born with but *acquired.* This way of doing things has been *repeated* so many times that it is performed easily and *automatically*, without conscious thought. Acting without conscious thought can be extremely helpful in everyday life. Having to think consciously about firing every nerve and moving each muscle to get out of bed or digest our food would leave us little time for anything else. If a particular habit is serving your spiritual nature as a joyful, willing, loving, healthy human being, by all means keep the habit. However, if a habit is contributing to ill health, unhappiness, self-hate, or hate of others, it may be time to replace that habit.

To replace a habit that is no longer useful with one that supports a healthy body, mind, and spirit, examine why that habit was acquired in the first place. Let's say, for example, that Sue has a habit of having a big breakfast every single morning. She gets up, gets out the eggs, toast, juice, and bacon, and begins cooking, without a conscious thought. She may have begun this habit at any time and for any reason. Maybe as a child she had a big breakfast every day. Her mother cooked it for her, and she sat down every morning with her family to eat before she left for school. Maybe her mother and her teacher always said, "Breakfast is the most important meal of the day. You have to eat well in the morning to do well at school." Take Fred, for another example of the same habit. Fred never really ate a big breakfast until the summer he started working construction and found that if he didn't eat a big breakfast he didn't have enough energy to work until lunch. Whatever the reason, way back when these people began the habit, they experienced benefits from choosing a certain way to act. The benefits may have been emotional or physical, but they were benefits—positive, pleasurable reinforcement that caused them to repeat the actions over and over. After frequent and prolonged repetition, the actions became automatic; they became a habit. Both Sue and Fred could feel pleasure from the act whether they had a physical need for a large breakfast or not, rather like Pavlov's dog. If you asked them years later why they always ate such a big breakfast, they would probably say, "I don't know. I've always eaten a big breakfast."

Where Do Beliefs Come From?

Beliefs come from life experiences and from thoughts that are repeated so many times that the subconscious mind decides they are truth. When a conscious thought such as "I need a big breakfast to do well in school" or "I need a big breakfast so I can work until lunch" is repeated over and over, it gradually becomes accepted as truth. It becomes a part of our subconscious belief system, the system of values, attitudes, and perceptions that we base our actions on. When we were born, our mind was a blank slate; we had no belief system. This allowed us to act through instinct and our true spiritual nature. Over the years, however, we acquired hundreds and thousands of subconscious beliefs. These beliefs are now the filter through which we view life. They are the foundation for our thoughts, actions, and reactions. We no longer operate on a moment-to-moment basis out of our natural instincts. We operate out of our acquired belief system.

Some of these beliefs are healthy and helpful—they support our instincts and our spiritual self. However, a great many of these beliefs are negative and do not support our true nature. This becomes quite apparent when we decide to change ourselves in some way and we can't seem to do it, no matter how hard we try. Very simply put, life experiences create our beliefs, out of these beliefs come our everyday thoughts, and from these thoughts arise our actions. Actions that are repeated over and over become habits.

Life Experiences → Beliefs → Thoughts → Actions → Habits

It is important to understand this cascade of events. We can't change the life experiences we have already had, but we can change our beliefs about them. The belief → thought → action → habit cascade is the backbone of change. Most popular literature says that if you just buckle down and perform a new habit for 21 days, it will be yours permanently. We have not found this to be true. In fact, people find it extremely difficult to get through the 21 days. This difficulty arises because we are trying to change an action without changing any of the underlying beliefs and thoughts that support it.

Having knowledge of or insight into a habit does not necessarily mean that you have changed the beliefs that support the habit. For instance, you may totally understand the benefits of drinking eight glasses of water a day. In fact you may even be a nutritionist who teaches people why they should drink water. But if you believe you can't possibly drink that much water, or water isn't satisfying or water tastes bad, you will never drink eight glasses of water a day, no matter what your knowledge level. You can force yourself to drink the water for a while, but the conflict between what you are *doing* and what you *believe* will become so uncomfortable that, as a pleasure-seeking being, you will abandon the water to preserve your peace and happiness.

Examine the beliefs you have that support your old habits. Then determine what beliefs you need to replace to provide a foundation for your new habits. Then start changing your beliefs! We will explain techniques you can use to change your beliefs in Chapter 17.

There is another aspect of habit formation that is equally important to know about when making changes. We create and/or maintain most habits to answer a need. Just breaking a habit without fulfilling the need in some other way will result in a return to the old habit or development of a new habit that may be better or worse than the original one. A classic example of this is the smoker who uses cigarettes to relieve stress. He decides to quit smoking, without any conscious thought he begins eating to relieve stress, and he gains 30 pounds. This occurs because when he quit smoking he addressed only the habit and not the need it was fulfilling.

Let's take a look at our big-breakfast scenarios. It is possible that Sue's big breakfast was meeting the physical needs of a growing child and inadvertently became associated with meeting emotional needs. Sitting down with her family and connecting with them before the day started gave Sue feelings of connection and love. As Sue grew up, she may have lost the physical need for a large breakfast, but if she was needy in the areas of love and connection, she may have held on to this habit to assist her in meeting those emotional needs. Habitually using food to meet emotional needs can lead to weight gain, but unless those emotional needs are met in some other way, giving up the food is extremely difficult.

The same sort of thing might occur with Fred, the construction worker. While he's working construction his habit of eating a large breakfast serves him well. He feels good, he works hard all the way until lunch, and he maintains a healthy weight. But suppose by some sort of accident he becomes disabled and takes on a desk job. His life is turned upside down. Eating a big breakfast every morning is something he has always done, and heaven knows he could use some order and predictability in his life. So he chooses to keep this habit, even though physically he is no longer doing a job that requires that kind of a breakfast. Eventually he may start to gain weight. However, unless he meets that need for order and predictability in his life in some other way, breaking the big-breakfast habit will be hard.

Replacing a habit involves three steps: (1) changing the subconscious beliefs that are supporting the habit; (2) determining the needs that a habit is filling and meeting those needs in some other way; and (3) developing a clear mental picture of yourself performing the new habit you desire. We often say human beings are creatures of habit. This may be true and necessary for certain physical functions, but nowhere is it said that we should live the majority of life by habit. That would mean living it unconsciously, automatically, and without thought. We have the freedom of choice. At any time we can choose to examine our habits and determine what they are doing for us and why. If your habits are not congruent with your true spiritual nature, it may be time for a change.

Opportunities for Growth

Awareness

- What things do you do by habit, automatically, without conscious thought? Make a list.

- Which of these habits support your health, happiness, and self-esteem? Which ones undermine your health, happiness, and self-esteem?

Introspection

- Can you trace any of the habits that are undermining your health or happiness back to the life experiences that created them?

- What does each one of the undermining habits you listed do for you? What comfort or avoidance of discomfort does it provide for you? You wouldn't keep these habits if they didn't do something for you.

- What are some of the beliefs you have that support these habits?

Old Beliefs to Let Go

- Habits are hard to break.

- I don't need to _____ [continue this habit]. I can stop anytime I want. I just don't want to.

- I'm not responsible for my habits.

- I can believe one way and act another way.

New Beliefs to Embrace

- My beliefs support my habits.

- Changing my beliefs provides the groundwork for easily changing my habits.

- I easily recognize the needs my habits are filling.

- I meet the needs my habits are filling in other, healthy, more nurturing ways.

Vividly Imagine

- Imagine what it would look like and feel like if you were able to think every minute like a naturally slim person. What would your new habits look like? What things would you be doing automatically? Imagine yourself meeting your needs for relaxation and joy without food. What would you be doing instead?

Patterns for Action

- Identify one small habit that is undermining your progress that you would like to change. Take that habit and trace it back to its origins.

• Identify the needs that this habit fills. What are the positive results of having this habit? What are the negative results? When did you begin this habit? What was going on in your life at that time? Do you still have the need that the habit was originally adopted to fill? If not, recognize that. If so, is there a healthier way to fill the need?

• Write down some new thoughts or beliefs that would support a change in this habit.

• Visualize yourself performing your new habit every day.

FIFTEEN

How Your Belief System Affects Your Life

Allow yourself to get distracted by living. There is a lot to be learned when your weight stops being the focus of your life.

AS CHILDREN WE START out totally in touch with our spirit, our true selves. We believe we can do anything and have an inward drive toward knowledge and growth. Our spontaneity, our self-love, our capacity for joy and wonder are unbounded. We are beautiful blank slates on which life's experiences, good and bad, etch new beliefs. Some sources say that the majority of the beliefs that form our overall perception of the world are in place by the time we are three years old. Whether or not this is true, by the time we reach adulthood our beliefs probably number in the hundreds of thousands. It is sad to note that a large portion of those beliefs are self-limiting and can stunt our personal growth. That is, instead of supporting the spirited joy and love of childhood, our adult beliefs shroud it with limitations, guilt, and fear. The spontaneous joy and happiness we possessed as children may be buried so deeply under negative beliefs that we cannot even feel their presence. If they do happen to break through on occasion, we are caught off guard, frightened, even embarrassed.

Our beliefs form the perceptions through which we view the world. Have you ever sat in a crowd and focused your mind on the color red? It is absolutely amazing how many red shirts, red hats, and red jackets you will see. Yet, if you change your predominant thought to blue, you begin to notice how very many blue hats and blue jackets there are. Have you ever bought a new car and then noticed in the next several weeks as you drive around town that everyone seems to have gone out and bought the exact same car? Of course this isn't true. All those cars were out there before; it is just that your perception has changed.

A belief, whether positive or negative, directly affects your perceptions of yourself and the world around you. It acts as a subconscious magnet and draws experiences to you that reinforce it. A belief put into action is very self-reinforcing. For instance, suppose you own the belief that you are unattractive. You will look at the world through the eyes of someone who is unattractive. You may be shy, avoid the opposite sex, walk with your head down, not dress well. Your whole demeanor will be affected by that belief, and indeed your physical and mental attitudes will keep people away from you. In turn you will say, "See, no one wants to be around me," and you will feel very justified in keeping that belief. Consequently you will keep attracting more and more experiences that reinforce it so that you continue to feel unattractive but right.

Beliefs in Everyday Life

Let's look at an example involving a relationship. Ellen has been married for 14 years. She loves her husband, but she's having a difficult time communicating with him. "I don't know . . . he is just not as well-read as I am, and sometimes the things he says are so stupid, so redneck, that I just get furious." Ellen can't change her husband, but she can change her own beliefs and perceptions about him. This is the list of beliefs I hear in that one single sentence:

My husband says stupid things.

My husband is stupid.

My husband isn't well-read.

My husband isn't as smart as I am.

My husband makes me furious.

As long as Ellen walks around with those beliefs, any time her husband makes a silly comment it will stick out like a red flag. Her mind is primed and ready and actually attracting those comments. Her husband may even get a charge out of her reactions, but that is his problem. Suppose that Ellen changed those beliefs to these:

My husband is bright and well-read.

My husband's comments are entertaining.

My husband is OK just the way he is.

Suppose that deep in her subconscious mind she truly believed these statements. Her perception of events with her husband would be entirely different, and the outcomes of their conversations would be also.

Jim has a job in a factory, working near a machine that makes a squeaking sound every 15 minutes or so. It has become very annoying to Jim. In fact he can almost feel his blood pressure rise every time it squeaks. Sometimes he even thinks about it before he gets to work! The squeak is part of the machine and cannot be changed, and Jim really doesn't want to look for a new job. What Jim can do is change his perception of the squeak. Right now he believes the squeak is loud, the squeak is annoying, he can't work well with the squeak, and the squeak is giving him a headache. Suppose he believed instead that the machine squeaks because it is doing a good job, the squeak is just background noise at a job that he likes, he is rarely annoyed by noises, and he is relaxed in the presence of noises. Any one of these would help tremendously to get that squeak into perspective rather than letting it dominate his life. What we believe affects absolutely every area of our lives—not just our weight and our health but also all of our relationships and our sense of self-worth.

Beliefs, Life, and Weight

The 10 habits of naturally slim people are about life, not just eating. That is what makes them both different and practical. This entire section of the book, addressing belief, thought, and habit changes, can be used in any area of your life, not just in your quest for health and slimness. Be OK with that. Allow the quality of your life to take precedence over the percent body fat you have. In the long run both your life and your figure will improve.

When Robin decided that she would never diet again and joined our classes, she had many things going on in her life, and she was 70 pounds overweight. She was a very unhappy person, and like many of us she thought if she "just lost some weight" she would "feel" better. Because we were teaching the importance of self-esteem in becoming slim, Robin chose to work daily on changing beliefs about herself and her worth. After about a month or two, Robin stopped coming to class. When we spoke to her, we found that she was still working on her personal growth but that she had gotten drawn away from her issues with food into her need to be needed by other people and how that was affecting her life. She started reading books on codependence, Ayurvedic philosophy, happiness, and self-love.

Robin spent a whole year discovering how she thought and what beliefs were leading to unhappiness in her life. When she returned to class after one and a half years, she was a much happier person. Her habit of eating to soothe her emotions had been altered significantly. Without even thinking about it, she had lost a dress size even though her weight remained the same. This meant she was experiencing a natural loss of fat and a healthy increase in muscle, the only way you can change your dress size permanently. Robin has continued with us and is now working more closely on her beliefs about food and exercise. She has lost 40 pounds.

When we ask people, "Why do you want to lose weight?" the responses overwhelmingly refer to feelings: they want to be healthy, to be happy, to feel better and more energetic. These kinds of feelings do not come from body size; they come from total life experience. We all know very slim people whose lives are a mess. They offer proof that being slim is not the answer to life's problems. We are telling you these stories because we want you to be OK with getting sidetracked from your weight by life. When you do, you are not really getting sidetracked; you are in the mainstream. Remember, the current shape of your body is a reflection of how you've been living your life. When you work on improving your life, you will always in some way be improving your body.

You are a complex individual. If you isolate your efforts to lose weight from your relationships with friends and family, the work you do, and the feelings you have about other aspects of your life, you will not be successful. This is one of the reasons weight loss programs fail 98 percent of the time. They tell you what to do without considering your unique physical, mental, and spiritual attributes as well as your lifestyle and life priorities. We applaud people who have fallen off the diet wagon because it shows the strength of their inner selves. It proves that they do have a sense of self and are not robots.

Don't set goals by the scale or the calendar. You will know when you've reached your goals by how you feel. Happier? Healthier? Better than you used to? If your goal when you picked up this book was to lose 50 pounds by a certain date, we hope you have changed your mind. We hope you have an ongoing goal to know and love yourself in body, mind, and spirit and to be in balance as you grow into a healthy, naturally slim body.

Looking at your entire belief system, rather than just your beliefs about food and fat, may become part of your journey to natural slimness. What's important is to choose to grow every day, no matter what area of your life you are focusing on. Mental and spiritual growth support physical health, and physical growth supports mental and spiritual health. Balance is essential. Focusing all your moments for days, months, or years at a time on food and exercise is not balanced living. I must warn you, however, that when body size, fat grams, food, and exercise regimes are dropped from your every-moment consciousness, you'll need to arm yourself with new lunchtime conversation.

Hunger, satisfaction, and a naturally slim body are ours by nature. Believe it and develop the mental images to make it happen.

Additional Reading

Bristol, Claude. *The Magic of Believing*. New York: Simon and Schuster, 1994.

Dewey, Barbara. *As You Believe*. Self-published. To order, call (415) 669-1664.

Dyer, Wayne, Ph.D. *You'll See It When You Believe It*. New York: Avon Books, 1989.

SIXTEEN

Detecting Beliefs That Sabotage Your Growth

"Why don't I do the things I say I want to do?"
The answer is in your subconscious beliefs.
Learn how to detect these sabotaging beliefs
and how you can change them.

OVER THE LAST five years we have not only studied the thoughts and beliefs of naturally slim people but have also come to know intimately the thoughts and beliefs of overweight people, especially chronic dieters. We have gathered this information from clients as well as our own experiences. Despite the sincere declarations of the desire to become slim, the amount of mental self-sabotage that we uncovered was amazing. Most overweight people harbor self-defeating beliefs like "Being slim is frightening," and "My fat protects me," or "I can never be satisfied with average amounts of healthy food," to name just a few.

Before you can change what you believe and start thinking and acting like a slim person, you must be aware of what you are thinking and believing now that keeps you overweight. Even the soundest, most nutritious, custom-tailored, health-producing eating and exercise suggestions will not be followed by people whose sub-conscious minds are filled with negative, self-limiting beliefs. There are several ways by which you can discover some of the beliefs that are sabotaging your efforts to become healthy and less fat. The ones we use most often are mirror work and muscle testing.

Mirror Work

It is said that the eyes are the windows to the soul. How many of us have recognized this as we gazed into the eyes of a loved one? Yet how many times have you gazed into your own eyes? When you look in the mirror, you look at your teeth, your hair, your nose, or where to put your eye makeup, but how often do you look directly into your own eyes, directly into your own soul? Not often, I'll bet. In fact we most purposefully avoid eye contact with ourselves, just as we might do with a stranger on the street. Gazing into the eyes of a person is an intimate gesture. We don't do it with just anyone. But is our self just anyone? This avoidance of eye contact with ourselves is a sign of how much we are a stranger to ourselves, how much we operate externally without reference to ourselves. Because we are strangers to ourselves and our own instincts, we get ourselves in trouble, like becoming obese.

Start your trip to becoming naturally slim by becoming acquainted with the person who wants to be slim—you! As you stand in front of the mirror looking into your own eyes, what are you feeling? What are you thinking? This exercise can give you powerful information about how you truly feel about yourself. Are you thinking about how ugly you look or how fat you are? Are you criticizing yourself? This is an indication that you need to work on your self-esteem. Next, start to talk to yourself. Take one of the 10 habits and act as if you own it. Say right into your own eyes: "I love myself" or "I eat only when I'm hungry." When you say these things, what do you feel? What does your heart say to you? Does it say things like, "*Not*" or "No way" or "Like hell you do"? This lets you know quite clearly that you do not believe what you are saying. Try saying, "I really and truly want to lose this excess body fat" and listen closely for that tiny voice in your heart. You might be quite surprised to find that it is saying, "No, you don't."

It is also very common for overweight people to avoid looking at their bodies in the mirror. One of the reasons for this avoidance may be denial that they have a serious health issue to work on. The biggest reason, however, is that they cannot stand the constant onslaught of degrading thoughts they have about themselves. Avoiding the mirror is an act of self-preservation for these people. Others will look at themselves in the mirror and wallow in their negative thoughts, hoping it will shame them into action. It is a fact, though, that shame and punishment are very poor motivators for change. Lasting changes are made out of love and true concern for one's own well-being. Criticizing yourself and hating your body will not get you where you want to go, especially if what you want is to be naturally slim. If you hate your body, why would you want to take care of it by feeding it healthy foods or going for a walk? If you hate your body, why would you trust it to tell you when it is hungry and satisfied?

Use your mirror. Look directly at yourself and listen to what you are saying in your mind. Write it down and start to change it. If all you can hear are negative thoughts, look at just your eyes, just your hair, or some other part of your body that you accept and say so to yourself. Gradually move to another part of your body, one finger at a time if you have to, and begin to accept yourself. Look at that finger or arm or leg and marvel at the work it does for you every day. Marvel at how you can trust it to respond to your every whim. Every part of your body is truly a miracle. The size is merely a temporary result of not loving yourself enough. Forgive yourself for that, know that things can be different, and move on in your growth.

Use your mirror to gaze into your soul and find the truths about what you believe. Gaze into your eyes, make any statement you want about yourself or the way you eat, say it with feeling and conviction, then listen for a response from your subconscious mind. Do you truly believe what you are saying? Sometimes we have found when it comes to a positive loving statement about ourselves that we can't even get the words out or we start crying. That is a very vivid indication that you do not believe what you are saying and that you are very, very sad that you do not. Stay with those tears, cry them out, and when you are finished, ask what you can do for yourself to make things better. You can use the list of belief statements at the end of any chapter or make up your own using the guidelines in Chapter 17.

Self-Talk

When we first started working with clients, one of our primary goals was to help them turn around their negative thinking. We felt if we could help them get their thoughts changed around, it would be easier for them to begin to follow their instincts. So we asked them to write down the negative thoughts and feelings they experienced as they looked into the mirror or at other times of the day. We then asked them to take each negative thought and rewrite it as a positive thought, or affirmation, and to say that to themselves many, many times throughout the day, to create what some people call *positive self-talk*.

What we found out is that positive self-talk is definitely more supportive than negative self-talk, but that its ability to cause behavior changes was almost nil. People resisted doing affirmations, and it turned out that saying them more than two or three times a day became self-defeating. Why *would* you ever say anything to yourself 10 or 20 times a day unless you doubted it could be true? Saying the affirmations over and over therefore often increased disbelief instead of lessening it.

That is because when you say one thing and believe another, all you do is create mental conflict. Your mind-body-spirit system is always moving toward balance and conflict resolution. Consequently affirmations that are not supported by beliefs are soon abandoned. Self-talk occurs in the conscious mind, but we have discovered that changing a conscious thought does not support permanent behavior changes *unless* the thought change is supported by a change in *subconscious* beliefs. It is your subconscious beliefs that are your truth detector or your touchstone for your self-talk. When that little voice says, "*Not,*" it is your subconscious making the truth known to you.

This is not to say it's impossible to change a belief with self-talk. It can be done, but it takes much time and persistence and is usually extremely uncomfortable—it is called *brainwashing*. A much more pleasant and user-friendly way to change beliefs is a technique called *psychological kinesiology*, which we will discuss in the next chapter. When you change your beliefs, you begin to change your thoughts. When your thoughts are changed, the actions will follow.

Mirror work will provide you with some good information, but it relies on your ability to hear that little subconscious voice that evaluates the truth of what you are saying. Many people are unable or unwilling to hear that little voice. For this reason we recommend using a more reliable and objective method called *muscle testing*, which utilizes the complex neurochemical and electromagnetic system that exists between the mind and the body.

Mind and Body, Intimately Connected

Although we often speak of the conscious and subconscious mind as totally separate entities, it is important to understand that there is constant communication between the two levels. Every thought we think or action we take consciously has already been filtered through and directed by the subconscious mind. Not only are the two levels of consciousness constantly communicating, but communication goes on constantly between your mind and body as well. Even during sleep the mind-body system is alive with neurochemical and electromagnetic messages.

If you remember a little of high school chemistry, even the very tiniest molecule of your body is held together by the interaction and magnetic force of electrically charged atoms. The movement of fluid into and out of every cell in the body is also based on electrical charges. One aspect of this electrochemical communication system that is just beginning to be recognized by traditional science is the pervasive presence of neuropeptides and receptor sites outside the brain. Every word you utter, indeed every thought you think, releases millions of packets of neurochemicals that bathe not just your mind but every cell in your body. This is how stress causes stomach ulcers and why "type A personalities" are prone to heart attacks. When you find yourself in a life-threatening situation, you can feel the neurochemicals affecting your heart rate, breathing, sweat glands, and skin. These are important biological responses that help you either run faster or fight harder when faced with danger.

Even though you are not physically in a dangerous situation right now, close your eyes and vividly imagine that you are. Imagine a huge hairy poisonous spider crawling up your leg. Feel the hairs prickling and the eight tiny feet inching their way up to your soft, vulnerable abdomen. You scream but nothing comes out . . . Continue this vivid imagination and you will find you get the same physical response as you would if it were really happening. Your heart pounds, your skin crawls, you may perspire, or your knees may shake. All of this is caused by a thought.

All day long, to a lesser degree, what you think causes various physiological reactions. You may notice them if they are large enough, or you may be so used to not paying attention that these physical sensations go unnoticed—that is, until they become severe enough to grab your attention with a headache, an ulcer, or a heart attack. Even then you usually reach for an aspirin or call a doctor instead of trying to figure out what you might have been doing to cause your body's "dis-*ease*."

Conflict, negative thoughts, unhappiness, and thinking or acting in ways that are incongruent with your true nature cause the release of stress-related chemicals. When your body is constantly barraged by these stress-response chemicals, it can cause physical disease. Conversely, laughter, exercise, meditation, hugs, or a walk in the park cause chemicals to be released that create a sense of well-being. These neurochemicals can assist the healing process.

Muscle Testing

Every physical act you perform is an absolute miracle. You do not have to consciously think of every step involved when you hold your arm out to the side. You have a conscious desire to hold it out, and your subconscious mind taps into an already-learned routine, sending a clear electrochemical message to the necessary muscles to do the work. Muscle testing taps into this subconscious part of the muscle contraction.

Muscle testing has been used for years in different health care disciplines, often to see if certain foods or medications cause physiologic conflict in a person's system. In psychological kinesiology, we use it to test for conflicts between a person's conscious, spoken beliefs and the beliefs that exist in the fabric of the subconscious mind. Muscle testing is a much more reliable method than mirror work for detecting beliefs that are sabotaging people.

During muscle testing the subject is asked to say a belief out loud and hold it in her mind while the strength of one of her muscles, usually the arm muscle, is tested. If there is agreement, or congruence, between her spoken statement and subconscious belief, the mind sends a clear, strong electrical message from the brain to the muscle being tested. The tester will feel a good strong contraction. If there is conflict between what the person is saying and what she believes, communication between the brain and the muscle is muddled, and the electrical signal to the muscle being tested is weakened. In this case the tester will feel a lack of strength in the muscle being tested. This response will occur even if the person being tested is an extremely muscular weight lifter.

How to Perform Muscle Testing

Let's take a step-by-step walk through the muscle-testing procedure with two fictional characters, Samantha (the subject) and Theresa (the tester). Imagine that these two friends have decided to work together on changing their belief systems to help them release their excess body fat. Samantha and Theresa get together once or twice a week and help each other with muscle testing.

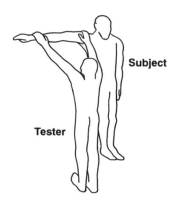

Figure 3. Muscle Testing

After a short chat, Samantha says to Theresa, "You know, I really think that I'm ready to lose all of this extra fat. I can't think of any reasons that I would want to keep it. Could you do some muscle testing with me to see if what I'm thinking is really true for my subconscious mind?" Theresa says, "Sure," and they proceed.

All that is necessary for a muscle-testing session is two willing participants, a pitcher of water and a glass, a pencil and paper for writing down belief statements and testing results, and a chair.

1. Samantha and Theresa stand face-to-face about a foot or so from each other. They close their eyes and take three deep breaths to gather their attention and to clear their minds for the task at hand.

2. Samantha and Theresa take turns, each stating their intention for being there. "It is my intention to participate in this muscle-testing session to assist myself and my partner in self-awareness and personal growth."
   These two steps set the stage for focused participation. Anytime muscle testing is used as a parlor trick or is attempted in distracting places or done in a hurry, the chances of obtaining inaccurate results are great.

3. Samantha drinks a few ounces of water.
   This step is important because our bodies are more than 70 per-

cent water. All electrical events, including the ones we are testing, occur more easily in a well-hydrated system. A subject who continually has weak muscle responses or is difficult to interpret during a muscle-testing session may need to drink more water.

4. Samantha chooses either her right or left arm to be tested and holds it out to the side, perpendicular to her body (see Figure 3).

5. Theresa stands facing Samantha, about a foot away, in front of the outstretched arm. She places one hand gently on Samantha's shoulder for stability and *gently* places her other hand on top of Samantha's outstretched arm, just above the wrist (see Figure 3).

6. Theresa asks Samantha to lower her eyes and look toward the floor. *This position of the eyes helps keep the subject associated with the emotions elicited by what she is saying. Looking forward or up in the air allows her to disassociate from what she is saying and can give inaccurate results.*

7. Theresa gives Samantha the testing instructions: "To become familiar with your muscles and how they test, I am going to ask you to do a few trials with me before we test the beliefs you wrote down. I will ask you to look down and repeat a statement for me. Immediately after you say the statement I will say, 'Be strong' and push down gently on your wrist for about two seconds. When I say, 'Be strong,' I want you to contract your shoulder muscle and resist my downward pressure while still focusing on the statement you have made.

   "Be sure to say the statement with feeling and conviction, and don't make any extra effort to fight against my downward pressure; just contract your muscle and resist.

   "Do you have any questions?"

   Samantha says, "No."

   It is important that the subject and the tester remain completely objective and curious about the results of the muscle test. Thinking, I'll bet this is true. This can't be false, muddles the electrical signals and can influence the results of the test.

8. Theresa gives Samantha a statement she knows is true, such as "My name is Samantha." Samantha repeats the statement with feeling, and Theresa says, "Be strong" and presses down gently on Samantha's wrist for about two seconds.
   Because the statement is true and congruous, the electrical signal to the muscle will be strong and Theresa will feel a strong muscle response.

9. Next, Theresa gives Sam a statement to make that she knows is false, such as "My name is George." Samantha repeats the statement, eyes down, with strong conviction, and Theresa says, "Be strong" and presses down on Samantha's wrist gently for about two seconds.
   Because the statement is false, it will cause conflict in Samantha's subconscious mind. This will weaken the signal to her shoulder muscle, and Theresa will feel a weakened muscle response. The muscle may waver, go soft, and then try to regroup, or Samantha's arm may drop completely down to her side. This proves that what Samantha was consciously saying, even with the strongest of convictions, was not true when run through her subconscious belief system.
   A strong muscle response indicates congruence, truth, or yes. A weakened muscle response indicates conflict, untruth, or no.

   This preliminary testing of known truths provides the tester with some practice sessions to become familiar with each new subject's muscle responses, and it allows the subject to get comfortable with the testing procedures and to trust the results. Now Samantha and Theresa are ready to test any belief statement they want.

10. Samantha says, "I'd like to test the statement 'It is important to me to remain fat.'" Theresa and Samantha follow the preceding procedure, with Samantha saying the statement she has chosen. Samantha says the statement, then Theresa tests the muscle response and finds it to be strong—just as strong and sure as when Samantha said her own name.

Wow, what a revelation! According to this muscle test, Samantha truly believes, in her subconscious mind, that it is important to remain fat. She was not aware of this consciously. Just imagine how a belief like this could cause her to continuously sabotage herself every time she tries to change the way she eats.

During the session Samantha and Theresa may change roles so that Theresa can test some of her beliefs. Maybe Theresa will find out that she believes nutritious food can never be satisfying or that she hates shopping, so she never has healthy food available in her house. Couldn't these beliefs also sabotage any efforts Theresa might be making toward health and slimness?

There are hundreds of beliefs that affect your health, your relationships, your prosperity, and most important, your openness to trying new things and your willingness to change and grow. Do you believe that change is hard? Do you believe that no matter what you do you will never be slim? Do you believe it is your destiny to remain fat? Do you believe fruits and vegetables are awful? Use mirror work or have a partner test you for the beliefs in the "Opportunities for Growth" section at the end of each chapter. Make up some belief statements of your own; there are guidelines for writing belief statements in Chapter 17.

Anyone with a genuine desire can learn to do muscle testing. As with almost any new technique, the better you understand it and the more you practice it, the easier it becomes. At the end of Chapter 17 there is information on where to obtain a videotape that presents the muscle-testing process. Clear your mental path, believe that you can do muscle testing, team up with a friend, and practice. If you find that you are not ready to learn or practice muscle testing right now, that is OK. Don't abandon the naturally slim process. You can use mirror work and maybe go to a workshop or get a videotape to help you learn muscle testing when you are ready.

Beliefs That Keep You Fat

We know it is hard to believe that you want to stay fat when you've been working so hard to get slim. You have had to work so hard because you have been working against yourself. The truth is that food and fat have been filling one or a number of needs for you. Once you discover what your beliefs about being fat are, you can change them and begin to meet those needs differently.

The following beliefs were gathered from overweight people attending our workshops. Some of them may or may not belong to you. You can use muscle testing to find out. My extra fat . . .

keeps me warm.

is like a continuous hug.

makes me different.

gets me noticed.

makes me feel large, more powerful.

protects me.

makes me feel safe.

sets boundaries for me.

keeps men away.

makes people expect less of me.

lets me expect less of myself.

keeps me from feeling small and vulnerable.

is like a security blanket.

means I can eat more.

means I can use food for love and comfort.

makes me visible.

Opportunities for Growth

Awareness

- Mirror-test or muscle-test the beliefs just listed. Keep a record of your beliefs.

Introspection

- Sit quietly or in whole-brain posture (Chapter 17) and ask yourself, "What does my extra body fat do for me?" Write down whatever comes into your head, no matter how crazy it may seem to you. Have a friend muscle-test these beliefs for you, or use the mirror test.

Old Beliefs to Let Go

These are all of the beliefs that keep you overweight, including the ones from your introspection. Also:

- I can't stand to look at myself in the mirror.

- I can't hear an inner voice when I do mirror work.

- Muscle testing is too hard to learn.

- I don't know anyone who would learn muscle testing with me.

New Beliefs to Embrace

- I am ready, willing, and able to hear my inner voice now.

- I enjoy doing mirror work, and I appreciate the insights it gives me.

- I am willing to learn muscle testing.

- Learning muscle testing is easy and enjoyable.

Also rewrite all the beliefs that keep you fat into present-tense positive statements that support the release of your excess fat.

Vividly Imagine

- Reread the mirror work section and the muscle-testing process. Build an image of yourself doing both—first doing mirror work, then finding a friend and doing muscle testing. Build the setting, including the kinds of things you are saying. Be sure to include the feeling of being OK with what you learn—surprised, amazed, but also appreciative of what you now know about yourself. Feel the empowerment of having a way to care for yourself and know yourself better. Visualizing this work will help dispel any fears you may have of the process or what you will find out.

Patterns for Action

- Find someone who will read this book at the same time you are and do muscle testing together on a regular basis.

- If you are uncomfortable with muscle testing, do mirror work for now, but make a commitment to get the videotape or attend a workshop to increase your comfort level. (See the end of Chapter 17 for information.)

Additional Reading

Diamond, John, M.D. *Your Body Doesn't Lie*. New York: Warner Books, 1979.

Levine, Barbara Hoberman. *Your Body Believes Every Word You Say*. Santa Rosa, CA: Aslan Publishing, 1991.

Using the Mind-Body Connection to Change Your Beliefs

"To change the printout of the body, you must learn to rewrite the software of the mind."

Deepak Chopra, M.D., in *Perfect Health*

NOW THAT YOU'VE taken the time to discover some of the self-limiting beliefs that you have, you probably have a desire to change some of those beliefs. Remember, it is your beliefs that create the way you think, and it is the way you think that creates your actions. Changing self-limiting beliefs to growth-enhancing beliefs provides you with a foundation for successful change.

In the past, change has been approached mostly from the outside in: self-talk, willpower, and "Just buckle down and do it." Now, however, we have techniques that can facilitate change from the inside out. The discipline of psychological kinesiology offers a series of techniques called *balances* that promote rapid changes in the program files of the subconscious mind. A balance can "delete" a negative subconscious belief you have had for decades and "add" a positive belief in a matter of minutes. This rapid shift is possible because balancing taps into the high-speed, whole-brain processing that we all have available to us.

Look at the clock and then close your eyes and imagine your last vacation. Quickly review in your mind what you did, the highlights of each day, and then open your eyes and look at the clock. How long did that take? Was it less than a minute? We can literally review our entire life in a nanosecond. Why shouldn't we be able to do a little subconscious reprogramming in the same length of time? In some ways our minds are very much like computers. Like a futuristic hard drive, the mind is wired for unlimited potential, and our subconscious beliefs are the software that is running continuously on the screen of our conscious mind, printing out the actions of our day-to-day life. To quote Rob Williams, founder of the Psych-K Centre in Denver, Colorado, "When you want to make changes, it makes a lot more sense to go in and change the software of your mind to change the printout of your life, rather than yelling at the printer. . . . The printer prints only exactly what the software program tells it to."

Right Brain + Left Brain = Whole Brain

Humans are blessed with the most advanced brain on the planet, and yet scientists estimate we use only about 2 percent of our brain's full potential. Just imagine what we could do if we harnessed even 1 percent more! Our brain is anatomically divided into two hemispheres: the right hemisphere and the left hemisphere. These hemispheres are connected by a bundle of fibers, kind of an information superhighway called the *corpus callosum*. Over the centuries of our evolution, this superhighway has been getting larger. Maybe someday we will all be able to think with our whole brain all the time. However, right now each hemisphere remains specialized, and most of us have a dominant hemisphere that prevails in the way in which we process information and solve problems:

Left Hemisphere	**Right Hemisphere**
• Language, reading and writing	• Visual-spatial relationships
• Thinks in words	• Thinks in pictures
• Utilizes logic	• Utilizes intuition, emotion, creativity
• Thinks linearly	• Thinks in whole and relation to part
• Thinks sequentially	
• Analyzes, breaks apart	• Thinks simultaneously
• Time aware	• Synthesizes, puts together
• Extroversion	• Time free
• Ordered	• Introversion
• Identifies with individual	• Spontaneous
	• Identifies with group

As you can see, each hemisphere complements the other, so it is to our advantage to be able to move back and forth easily between the two, and it is an even greater advantage to be able to operate out of both simultaneously. The EEG pattern of a person doing transcendental meditation shows equal activity in both hemispheres. It is conjectured that great inventors and artists such as Albert Einstein and Leonardo da Vinci were able to use both hemispheres equally well.

However, that still leaves us regular people who generally operate from one hemisphere or the other at any given moment. Sticking with one side of our brain when we are trying to problem-solve can lead us to be overly emotional or overly logical in our efforts. We may be able to visualize a solution but not be able to put it into words. We may be spontaneous and free and never come up with an answer to meet a deadline. Each hemisphere has its strength, but the two of them working together are synergistic and can accomplish the rapid processing that occurs with a psychological kinesiology balance.

What Is Psych-K?

Psychological kinesiology (Psych-K™) is a discipline developed by Robert M. Williams, M.A., a psychotherapist in Denver, Colorado. Psych-K uses kinesiology, or muscle testing, to identify subconscious beliefs that are limiting a person's potential for growth and change. Once a limiting belief is identified, a step-by-step process called a Psych-K balance is used to change this belief from a negative force to a positive force on which a person can build new behaviors. When a Psych-K balance is completed, you experience immediate feedback on the success of the belief change through post-balance muscle testing. According to Rob Williams, Psych-K is a "user friendly way to dissolve resistance to change."

Each Psych-K balance is designed to access both hemispheres of the brain simultaneously, through body posture or body movements. When a new idea or belief is introduced in a "whole-brain" state, that belief is easily assimilated into the subconscious mind. Although there are several different Psych-K balances, we will be introducing you to the whole-brain posture in this book. The whole-brain posture can be used as a stress-release tool and a belief-change balance. So, even if you are not ready to do any belief-change balances, take some time to learn the whole-brain posture and how to use it for stress release.

The Whole-Brain Posture

Two additional major roles of the brain are control of motor function and proprioception, the continuous awareness of where all of the body parts are at any given moment. The right hemisphere of the brain is in charge of the motor function and proprioception of the left side of the body, and the left hemisphere of the brain is in charge of those functions for the right side of the body. By sitting in a posture where your arms and legs cross the midline of your body and the right side and left side of your body touch in many places, both hemispheres become activated (see Figure 4). As we mentioned earlier, having access to both sides

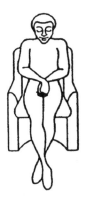

Figure 4. Whole-Brain Posture

of the brain simultaneously gives us the ability to see, hear, feel, and problem-solve in an entirely different way.

The first time you use whole-brain posture, you will need to determine your "optimal" position (right over left or left over right). You can determine this by having someone muscle-test you or, if no one is available, you can try both positions and feel the difference as described following the directions.

Here are step-by-step instructions for sitting in the whole-brain posture:

1. Sit comfortably in a chair with your right ankle over your left and have a partner muscle-test you. In this instance, the muscle test can be performed while seated and without any statement. If the test is strong, your optimal position is right over left from now on. If the test is weak, try left over right. If that is strong then your "optimal" position is left over right from now on.

    If you have no one to muscle-test you, use right over left and follow the rest of the directions. After you're in whole-brain posture, follow the asterisked directions for determining your optimal position.

2. Cross your ankles in your optimal position.

3. Put both arms straight out in front of you, palms down.

4. Keeping your palms down, cross one wrist over the other. Cross right over left if your ankles are right over left. Cross left over right if your ankles are left over right.

5. With your wrists crossed, move your palms downward and toward each other until they meet and fold your fingers together.

6. You can place your crossed, folded hands in your lap as in Figure 4, or you can turn them inward toward your chest and rest them on your breastbone. You are now in whole-brain posture. *If you were not muscle-tested for your optimal position, sit in whole-brain posture quietly as you are now, right over left, and clear your head. Whole-brain posture should be relaxing, quiet, and nonstressful. After you sit for a few minutes, switch your position to left over right and sit quietly again, noting whether you feel relaxed or tense, agitated or calm. Your optimal position is the one you feel most mentally relaxed in. It has nothing to do with whether you usually cross your legs one way or the other. When you determine your optimal position, write it down for future use.*

Whole-Brain Posture as a Stress Reducer

Now that you know how to do the whole-brain posture, you will find a million uses for it. Throughout our days we come across many situations that trap us into one side or another of our brain. We get either overly emotional or overly logical in arguments with family and coworkers, or we sit in a meeting that is long and boring and are extremely anxious about getting out. We are stressed; we look at a piece of food that we want to eat. We're not even hungry, and we eat it anyway (not too logical, right?). When you find yourself in any of these situations, notice how tense and stressed you are. Take a deep breath and sit in whole-brain posture. You can actually feel the stress dissolve. What is especially great is that you can sit in whole-brain posture anytime, anywhere, and people won't even notice. On an airplane or a bus, in court, at the dinner table, or in class, it is a wonderful tool.

Whole-brain posture can also be very useful in providing you with a balanced self-perspective when you are doing the introspection exercises in this book. Try doing your thinking in whole-brain posture.

Whole-Brain Posture as a Balance for Belief Changes

The whole-brain posture can be used specifically to incorporate new subconscious beliefs into your life. For the first time you can feel empowered to build your health from the inside out. You can build a foundation for change by reprogramming your own subconscious mind. The actual steps of the balance are as follows:

1. Choose a belief statement.

2. Muscle-test your belief statement.

3. Sit in whole-brain posture.

4. Allow belief-change processing to occur.

5. Lock in a new belief.

6. Muscle-test your belief statement.

    1. Choose a Belief Statement. Choose a belief statement that you would like to be a permanent part of your subconscious programming. You can choose a belief statement from anywhere in this book, or you can make up your own. If making up your own statement, write it down. Be sure to write it in the present tense, leave out negative statements, and state what you want, not what you don't want. A well-formed belief statement would be "I easily recognize my physical hunger signals"—it is present tense and positive. An unusable statement would be "I *will never* ignore my hunger signals"—it uses *will*, which denotes the future; it is negative; and it states what you don't want instead of what you do.

    2. Muscle-Test Your Belief Statement. After you've chosen or written the statement, have a friend muscle-test you following the procedure in Chapter 16. This will tell you whether you already believe the positive statement or not. If your muscle test is weak, you do not believe the statement and you can balance for it. If your muscle test is strong, choose a different belief to balance.

If you don't have anyone to do a muscle test, and you know you don't believe a statement because of mirror work you have done, you can still balance for the belief; you just won't have muscle-test verification of your results.

3. Sit in Whole-Brain Posture. Follow the six-step procedure for sitting in whole-brain posture. If you already know what your optimal position is, proceed to step 2.

4. Allow Belief-Change Processing to Occur. Once you are in whole-brain posture, be sure that you know the correct wording of your belief statement and close your eyes. Repeat silently to yourself, with all of your heart, the new belief that you want to make part of your subconscious mind. Keep repeating this statement silently and slowly to yourself and invite in any conflict or resistance associated with adopting this new belief.

What you are doing in this step is exposing your whole brain to a new belief, which it will store as a file in your subconscious mind. After the new file is installed, it will supersede your old belief file. To get the new belief filed, your subconscious has to sift through old files, old beliefs, old memories, and life experiences that might oppose this new belief. While you are sitting, silently repeating your belief statement, your subconscious mind will start processing very rapidly. During this processing you may experience any one or none of the following things: fluttering eyes, visual images, self-talk fighting the belief, tightening of the muscles of the face or whole body, tears, laughter, or other physical sensations. None of these sensations are right, and none of them are wrong. They are all individual to what your unique mind needs to process to assimilate the new belief into your system.

You will know when the process is finished because you will experience a subtle or not-so-subtle shift in your brain and/or your body. Some people have a dramatic shift from crying to peace to laughter. Some just feel the tension released from their head or

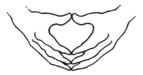

Figure 5. Lock in a New Belief

their arms; some people just feel a sense of comfort with what they are saying to themselves where before there was a sense of conflict. Just tune in to yourself and trust that you will know.

5. Lock in a New Belief. When you are finished processing, stop repeating your belief statement, open your eyes, uncross your legs and arms, and put your 10 fingertips together as shown in Figure 5. This is a physical signal to your brain to save the new program you have installed. Hold your fingers there for 10 to 15 seconds and just feel how at peace you are.

6. Muscle-Test Your Belief Statement. Stand up and say your new belief while your partner muscle-tests you. Your response should be very strong, because now what you are saying with your conscious mind is in complete agreement with your subconscious beliefs. If you test weak, take a sip of water and test again. If the muscle response is still weak, the balance is not complete. Go back into whole-brain posture and repeat the balance until the processing is complete and the muscle test is strong.

Balances and Time

There is no average length of time that it takes to balance for a new belief. We have experienced 30-second balances and 45-minute balances. It all depends on what your subconscious has associated with that belief. Most balances take only a few minutes; don't be scared away by the time. If a balance is taking longer than 30 minutes, you may have too complicated a belief statement. Keep your statements simple. Don't put really big psychological issues into one balance. Try breaking them into smaller pieces. Don't balance using words that you don't understand. If you absolutely have to stop in the middle of a balance, you can return to it later, but you should start the balance over.

A balance lasts for as long as it is useful to you, which is usually for the rest of your life. However, if you and your life are growing and changing, there may be a time when your subconscious needs to refile a certain belief and you will test weak to a statement you already balanced. Just go ahead and balance on that statement again.

Exercising Your Potential

Our clients frequently ask, "When will I see myself change now that I have balanced for a new belief?" We'd love to be able to tell you that exactly 14 days after you balance on the statement "I am a concert pianist" you will be able to play the piano brilliantly, but it doesn't work that way. When you balance for a new belief, you clear a path, you remove obstacles, and you increase your potential. How soon that potential will be actualized depends on where you are and what you do with it. Some people have experienced profound changes in their lives after a Psych-K balance and nothing else. Others have left their beliefs dormant and never experienced any changes, and there are cases everywhere in between. Most people will report that they experience very subtle changes in their perceptions of things over the weeks following their balances. They notice little differences in things they say or do that surprise them because they are so unlike themselves.

We encourage people to support their new beliefs with vivid imagery—the more vivid, the better. Create a three-dimensional animated movie of yourself eating slowly, buying vegetables, looking slim in a bathing suit, walking outside, or manifesting whatever new belief you have balanced. Giving your conscious mind thoughts, patterns, and images to follow will shorten the time between belief change and behavior change (see "Framing,"

Chapter 18). Reading books, taking workshops, going to lectures on the principles you now believe in will increase the conscious knowledge base from which you operate. Remember, however, that just exposing yourself to knowledge does not guarantee change. You must have your belief system in place.

Where Should I Start?

Some of you may look at the instructions for whole-brain posture and say with a sigh, "It all seems too complicated." In that case you may want to balance for the beliefs "I easily understand Psych-K" and "I welcome changes in my life." Others may say, "I don't have time for all of this stuff," in which case you may want to balance for the belief "I always have time for personal growth work." The greatest gift you can give to yourself is time, on a daily basis, to pursue your personal growth. Most of us lead pretty hectic lives, and we're used to saying, "I don't have enough time." The answer is to work on Habit 1: get your life priorities straight, and you will find the time.

Some of you will be excited because now you have some tools to work with and you will be tempted to jump in and start changing every belief that you can think of, especially the ones that have to do with your weight. This is OK, but don't burn yourself out. Doing daily work in one area, reading a chapter, doing the exercises, doing some mirror work and some Psych-K, and building your vivid images can be more helpful than balancing for 100 new beliefs and never exercising any of their potential. Give yourself time; give yourself space; don't force yourself to use this book like a diet. Respect yourself and your feelings. If doing balances doesn't feel right to you, go through the book and find what does feel right. This book is about self-referral and choice. Listen to yourself and choose. You will always choose what is best for you whether it is just being peaceful with where you are or taking advantage of an opportunity to grow.

Opportunities for Growth

Awareness

- Sit in whole-brain posture and notice how you feel mentally.

Introspection

- Stop and think. How do you feel about the information you have been given in these last two chapters? This can seem like pretty radical stuff compared with the usual food plans and recipes found in most books about weight loss.

- Did any of your other adventures into weight loss books or programs work?

- Are you ready to try something new?

- Are you avoiding taking responsibility for your life and your weight? If so, why? Who else is going to take responsibility for them?

- If you have questions or doubts about muscle testing and Psych-K, are you willing to reread the chapters? Make a phone call and ask questions? Take a workshop or view a videotape?

Old Beliefs to Let Go

- Old dogs can't learn new tricks.

- I don't have the time to do/learn this stuff.

- I just need someone to tell me what to eat; not all this hocus-pocus.

- This is all too confusing.

New Beliefs to Embrace

- I am willing to learn and undertake new processes that enhance my health.

- I am a spirit inside a body, and I believe in the power of the mind-body connection to make me well.

- I learn new things easily and enjoy the practice it takes to be comfortable.

- I have all the time I need to foster my personal growth.

- I have confidence in muscle testing and balancing, and they are easy to learn.

Vividly Imagine

- Reread the step-by-step process for whole-brain posture and then imagine yourself doing it step-by-step.

Patterns for Action

- Dedicate one hour a day to personal growth.

- Practice whole-brain posture whenever and wherever you find yourself feeling stress.

- Once you get comfortable with using whole-brain posture for stress release, start doing belief-change balances and build your foundation for health one belief at a time.

Additional Reading

Dacher, Elliot, M.D. *PNI, Psycho-Neuroimmunology—The New Mind/Body Healing Program*. New York: Paragon House, 1991.
Russell, Peter. *The Brain Book*. New York: Plum, 1979.

For further information about upcoming Psych-K workshops, call or write to: The Psych-K Centre, 2055 S. Oneida St., Suite 350, Denver, CO 80224; (303) 756-9725.

To order videotapes on Psych-K by Rob Williams, call (800) USA-TAPES. Currently available: *Free Yourself from Limiting Beliefs*. This video demonstrates muscle testing and presents 12 self-esteem-supporting beliefs and a Psych-K balance.

EIGHTEEN

Three-Dimensional Nutrition: Food for the Spirit, the Mind, and the Body

The self has three inseparable dimensions: spirit, mind, and body. When we starve any one dimension, we starve the whole. When we lovingly nourish any one dimension, we nourish the whole.

PICTURE IN YOUR MIND a blank piece of paper with a single line representing one dimension. The line can stand or lie down and slant in an infinite number of ways. It has great potential but is somehow lacking in its totality. It yearns for a completeness that it cannot have if it remains a straight line in a single plane. However, when it turns a corner or two, it becomes two-dimensional. It has length and width, and its potential for becoming is increased. It can be a square, a circle, a parallelogram, a rhombus, a rectangle, a hexagon, an octagon, and more. However, it remains flat and somewhat lacking in vitality. Add to it a third dimension, depth, and it literally pops off the page and begins to dance. Length, width, and depth have value as separate entities, yet by themselves they are flat. Put them together, and the dynamics of the three create a vivid picture with a life of its own.

Look, Mom, I'm 3-D!

It is the same when we consider the dimensions of ourselves. We are bodies, yet a body without a mind or a spirit is rather boring, to say the least—and not much different from a carrot, some might say. We have a mind, but a mind cannot exist without a brain, which is part of the body. We are spirits. Yet a spirit without a mind or a body is no longer a human being, and we would have great difficulty interacting with the world around us on a daily basis. The truth is we are human beings, we do live on this earth, and we do have three dimensions: body, mind, and spirit. There is a dynamic relationship among our body, mind, and spirit, and that is what makes the human race unique. We are primarily a spirit—an energy force, a life force, a soul that is inhabiting a physical body. The mind acts as a medium between the spirit and the body. The clearer we can keep the mind, the more focused we are in the present moment, the less we worry and fret, and the easier it is for us to act physically like our true selves.

Each of our three dimensions is equally important, and all three interact with each other. Each of these dimensions has its own unique "nutritional" needs. Feeding one dimension in a healthy, loving manner affects the other dimensions indirectly. It is important to take the time to nourish and nurture all three. Thinking, experiencing, and feeling provide fuel for the mind and spirit. Learning how to think and how to change toxic thinking into nurturing thinking is as important as the food we put into our bodies. Most of us have spent a lot of time feeding and not feeding our bodies but have paid relatively little attention to feeding our minds and our spirits—not feeding them just anything but rather feeding them high-quality thoughts and ideas just as we strive to feed our bodies high-quality food. In the next few pages we will touch on the many ways there are to nourish all three dimensions of ourselves.

Nourishment for the Spirit

What Is a Spirit?

To feed the body in ways that produce health and slimness you must tend to feeding your spirit. You have spent years and decades studying calories and fat grams, abhorring celery sticks, and feeling guilty about the chocolate mousse you ate last night. You struggle endlessly to create a perfect physical body, and then, when you reach that perfection, it still doesn't feel right. Why? Because physical beauty really is only skin deep, and we all go much deeper than our skin.

Your physical body is only a vehicle for your wondrous spirit. Your spirit is who you truly are and has nothing to do with your religion. The spirit is referred to in many ways: it is your essence, your substance, the source of your creative self, your soul, your true self, your inner self, your higher self; the energy, the light, the spark that lights up your body and your mind and makes you who you are. I remember a story told by Wayne Dyer in which he speaks of his grandmother, who is terminally ill. They weighed his grandmother on a scale minutes before she died, and she was 150 pounds. As she quietly passed away, she was weighed a final time before they wrapped up her body. She was still 150 pounds. She still had all the physical attributes she had had moments ago, including her weight, but *she* was not there anymore.

How do we measure a spirit? Do we wait for scientists to prove we are spirits before we believe it? If we do, we will wait forever. When science dissects humanness down to its smallest subatomic particle, it ends up with pieces, physical, material pieces that never quite add up to a total human being. The sooner you can admit to yourself that you are more than just the sum of your physical parts, the sooner you can start feeding your spirit with spiritual food instead of table food. The sooner you stop feeding your spirit table food, the sooner you will hear your body's physical hunger and satiety signals and be able to release your excess body fat!

The Connection Between Spirit and Fat

Permanent loss of excess body fat occurs when the spirit, mind, and body are in dynamic equilibrium. Most of us are out of balance and have very little joy or peace in any of our three dimensions. So where should you start? Up until now most of you have been working diligently on your body to lose weight, and most of you have been unsuccessful. This time around, start with your spirit. Your spirit is your core, the inner supporting structure for who you are, and permanent change occurs from the inside out.

Sewing up the skin over a compound fracture of the leg without setting the bone leaves one with a leg that has no supporting structure, a leg that is painful and nonfunctioning, a leg that may temporarily look good on the outside but will begin festering and swelling until it bursts open and demands proper treatment. Pardon the graphic metaphor, but this is exactly what you do every time you try to fix your inner self by changing your outer fat layer. Think about all those times you worked so diligently on what you ate—how you exercised and you looked good on the outside for a while, and then it all seemed to fall apart. That was because you did not have the spiritual and mental infrastructure to support the physical changes. The continuous failure of your previous methods to produce the body you want indicates that the methods were faulty, not you. Healing must take place from the inside out. Your spirit and mind must begin to heal before you can manifest a healthy, slim body.

First Essential Nutrient: Pay Attention

The first step to spiritual nutrition is to recognize that you are more than a physical body, to consider the possibility that you have a soul, a higher self, or a spirit. Again, you do not have to be religious to do this. Whether you prefer the word *soul* or anything else doesn't really matter. What matters is that you believe you are more than a body and more than a mind. If you don't believe it, then what makes two genetically identical twins different? When you talk to yourself, who are you talking to? When you mull over things in your mind, who is the moderator? Who makes the choice? When you get an intuitive flash, when something touches your heart, where is this happening? When you are in love, who is in love? Your mind? Your body? What does it mean to have a friend who is a soulmate? Is life a beating heart? Breathing lungs? A functioning brain? I worked in an intensive care unit for many years. We could make a heart beat and lungs breathe, but when a person's spirit was gone there was not a thing we could do.

In Chapter 5 we talked about the qualities of your true self. Your spirit is that wonderful core of love, openness, willingness, and trust that showed through your eyes the day you were born. It is the spirit that we often forget to keep in touch with as our lives get more complicated and busy. It is loss of contact with this core that causes us stress, fear, and unhappiness. How can you tell when you are spiritually hungry? *Pay attention to your emotions.* It is inherent in our nature to be joyful, happy, healthy, loving, trusting human beings. When we do not feel this way—when we feel sad, depressed, fearful, hateful, angry, or unhappy—it is a signal that we are thinking and acting in ways that are not congruent with our true nature. Allow yourself to feel the feeling and then allow yourself to look beyond the feeling to its cause. Often that cause is spiritual hunger.

Paying attention is not just the first step toward nourishment of the spirit but also the most important step. Recognize that there is a part of you that desires some peace and quiet every day. Recognize that there is a part of you that longs to be in touch with nature, art, and music. Recognize that there is a part of you that sometimes wishes the rest of the world would go away and just leave you alone. Honor your need to be by yourself and do what you want to do. These are all messages from your spirit. It is reminding you that you are not just someone's spouse or someone's employee; you are not just someone's mother, father, son, or daughter. You are a unique individual in your own right, and you do need time by yourself, with yourself, getting to know your-self—time to think and fiddle around with hobbies, passions, and quests. Your spirit is your link to creativity. It is the gateway to being able to see each moment in life as an adventure, no matter where it takes you. When you see each phase of your life as an adventure and a learning experience, you open yourself to many more opportunities to experience happiness, joy, and fulfillment.

Meditation. Another way to pay attention to your inner self is to meditate. Some people have the mistaken impression that meditation is a religious practice, that it involves praying to God or recognizing Buddha or that it is against their religion if they are Catholics or Lutherans or any other denomination. Yes, some religions have forms of meditation in their practices, but medi-tation is not in and of itself religious. Meditation is not contem-plation or rumination, where you spend 30 minutes trying to figure out how to build a better mousetrap. In fact, in medita-tion you often reach a total absence of conscious thought.

A simplistic definition of meditation is the setting aside of time each day to sit in quiet with yourself as an observer of your own thoughts and then to gradually take attention away from your thoughts and sit in deep inner silence. Meditation allows you to release stress; it physically calms you and contributes to the improvement of many stress-related diseases such as high blood pressure. It allows you to experience the space between your thoughts, a gap in space and time where your spirit can surface, bringing you insight, intuition, creativity, and a sense of oneness with the universe. Many books and classes address various types of meditation. True to our philosophy of self-responsibility, we cannot say which type of meditation is best for you. You may want to try the following generic meditation:

Start out setting aside five minutes once or twice a day. Ded-icate this time to sitting in silence with yourself. Take the phone off the hook, sit down, close your eyes, and take three deep breaths. As you sit, many thoughts may float into your head—everything from what to make for supper to why you are sitting there. As these thoughts drift through, allow them to come and go without becoming attached to them. Don't get sucked into deciding what's for dinner. Let the thought go, or if you do get caught in it, recognize that you did and then let it go—no guilt, no right or wrong; it is just what it is.

Some people like to focus on a sound or their breath so they have a place to come back to when thoughts carry them away. Some days you will reach a state of silence and serenity easily; some days your mind will chatter incessantly; some days you will fall asleep. However the meditation goes, accept it for what it is and keep doing it. As this amount of time gets comfortable, increase the length of time to 10 minutes and then 15 minutes. Determine the length of time and number of times per day that are right for you.

When you meditate, choose a place that is relatively free from distractions. Some people choose a favorite chair, light a candle, and sit on a special mat or blanket. It is your meditation, so make up your own ritual. Rituals are very soothing to the spirit, mind, and body. Your meditation spot need not be totally silent. The dog may bark, the blinds may clatter, and that is OK. Part of a meditation can be being aware that there are sounds but not giving them attention. The purpose of this meditation is to take quiet time for yourself; to reconnect with your inner self and to release the stress and business of the mind. Meditation provides a time and a place for spirit to surface.

As you work with this minimeditation and increase your quiet time, begin to read about and experience other forms of meditation and see if they are right for you. Many of us work at home or at a job where the mere act of sitting down for a minute is construed as laziness ("sitting down on the job"). I recall many times when I fixed myself something to eat just so I had a legitimate reason to sit down and relax! We all need that kind of time. Give yourself permission to sit down and just *be* on a regular basis, whether you choose to meditate or not.

Music, Art, and Dance. We are energy! We are rhythm and pattern incarnate! The energy may be as quiet as one cell dividing to make new ones or as loud as a rock-and-roll drum solo. The rhythm may be as subtle as our breath during meditation or as noticeable as the dance moves we create to match those drums. It is because we are energy, rhythm, and pattern through and through that music, art, and dance can touch us so deeply. As our atoms, cells, and molecules vibrate, we search for similar vibrations to make us feel at home. Some people are touched by rhythm and blues, some by classical music. Some people are touched by Monet's paintings, some by a handmade quilt. Music and art are in the ears and eyes of the beholder. We all have music in us, and we all know how to dance. We can all create and appreciate art. Bring beauty into your life through music and art. Listen to different types of music. Find the ones that calm your scattered brain waves and the ones that make you smile and tap your feet. Look at different kinds of art and sculpture to find which ones touch your heart and which ones disturb you and make you think.

Once you have gotten comfortable listening and looking, be brave and think about doing. Even if it's playing a spoon against a glass, you may find an untapped source of joy when you take up a musical instrument, singing, dancing, or painting. Art, music, and dance existed long before written language. They are a part of our spiritual heritage and our relation to all human beings. Reach out for rhythms and patterns that cause you to feel, especially those that cause you to feel good and whole and connected.

Nature. Nature provides us with the supreme example of just being and growing, accepting life and accepting death as it comes. It is a place where we can literally feel rooted. We can walk among life in its simplest forms and learn lessons from the trees. Read the writings of Henry David Thoreau, who spent years learning about life from Walden Pond. Walking in nature also reminds us of how very little we need to experience the feeling of joy. Go outdoors and experience a sunrise, a flower, a blade of grass; the wind, the rain, the clouds. Fresh air, with or without sunshine, is nourishing to the soul. It is easy to get mindlessly caught up in the materialism of our society. We are continuously going, doing, striving for something better—a better house, a better job, a better body. The truth is, we all have absolutely everything we need right now. It is good to step back and question the direction your life is going in. It is your spirit that causes you to question.

The other great thing about nature (besides being free) is that trees, squirrels, and grass are totally nonjudgmental. They listen without interrupting, and they don't care how much you weigh. They radiate the same beauty in the presence of everyone, pauper or king. Gardening and working with the soil can be a very spiritual activity, as long as you aren't doing it because you "should" or "no one else will" or "it saves money." The mental attitude with which you approach any task will determine what you get out of it. The planting of seeds and the weeding, watering, and nurturing that cause them to grow are a great metaphor for your own process of growth and change. I have written an adult picture book based on this metaphor called *The Seeds of Change,* which I hope to have published soon.

Truth and beauty always vibrate at a level that touches the soul. All you have to do is be there!

"I'm Still Not Sure About This Spirit Stuff"

If as you read this you are still saying to yourself, "I really can't accept this spirit philosophy, but I'd still like to become naturally slim," understand that all of the principles about the mind and the body taught in this book are true, whether you believe in the concept of spirit or not. Many popular books and shows speak of the mind-body connection and play it safe by not mentioning the spirit. You will be able to succeed if you follow our suggestions, but without recognizing your true self it may be hard to look at these suggestions as anything different from a diet.

Our experience has been that when our clients believe they have an inner self or a spirit it is easier for them to love themselves even when they are very overweight, and self-love is absolutely essential to this process. Also, when clients admit to themselves that they are more than physical bodies and brains, they have a reference point for where they want to be as people rather than just wanting to "be slim." I found that in recognizing my true self I was much more able to feel deserving of good health and happiness and much more able to forgive myself and release guilt. If you are able to do all of these things easily, without believing you are a spirit, you will most likely be able to change your health and your weight permanently. Remember, your health and your weight are merely symptoms of the state of your life. When you work on your life in any sort of positive manner, you become much more able to improve your health and your weight.

Just as constant dieting may have caused you to disconnect from your physical hunger signals, constant spiritual starvation may have caused you to disconnect from your spiritual hunger signals. It is imperative that you begin feeding your spirit, whether it feels hungry or not. The key to spiritual nourishment is to be awake and aware and present in whatever activity you have chosen to do, whether it is a concert or a meal. Once you have mastered that, you will begin to realize that you can make absolutely anything spiritually nourishing, even scrubbing floors!

Nourishment for the Mind

We come into this world with a mind that is a blank slate. We spend the first half of our lives filling that slate with information and experiences both pleasurable and painful. We spend the second half of our lives erasing the slate and trying to figure out how to fill it with the truth. In our hearts, we somehow know that the truth will set us free, but we are not quite sure where to find it.

The mind works best when it is allowed to ebb and flow, with alternate periods of stimulation and rest. There is equal value in reading a book and doing meditation, taking a class and daydreaming, doing mental math and doing nothing. Always doing something with your mind and never doing anything with your mind are equally unbalanced. Notice that all the things that you do with a quiet mind, such as meditation, massage, listening to music, and looking at art, are activities that feed your spirit. Fill up your mind with thoughts that support life, love, liberty, and joy and then get out of your own way. As intelligent as human beings are, sometimes we really do think too much.

Feeding the Conscious Mind

What you are doing right now as you read this book is feeding your conscious mind. Exposing yourself to new information and ideas provides new perspectives through which you can create and view life experiences. We gather information through our five physical senses all day long, all the time receiving conscious information and weighing it against our established set of subconscious beliefs. Television, radio, movies, newspapers, books, audiotapes, magazines, and conversations add to our general sensory input.

It is important, whenever possible, to consciously choose your sensory input. Constantly exposing yourself to depressing accounts of crime, violence, and hate through the radio, television, and newspaper can take a toll on the types of thoughts and feelings you have. Surround yourself with healthy, positive, growth-oriented material. Skip the evening news once in a while and read the middle "life"-oriented section of your newspaper instead of the front page. Buy some of the books we have listed as recommended readings. Choose something new to learn, and exercise those brain cells. Most people begin to lose their mental powers as they age because they don't use them and they expect to lose them. There are wonderful books and tapes out there to help improve all your mental processes.

Fortunately, we do not retain every bit of sensory input we receive. If we did, we'd probably go crazy. Our mind filters what comes in and what is consciously acknowledged so that we don't "overload." You may have had the experience of sensory overload where there is so much stimulation coming into the brain that you literally can't think straight. This type of feeling can occur every minute of the day in children and adults with a nervous system that does not filter sensory information. For people with ADD (attention deficit disorder), who have low sensory thresholds, the ability to concentrate on a task while wearing itchy socks and sitting in a room with bright lights can be almost impossible.

Feeding the Subconscious Mind

Our subconscious mind acts like a magnet. It attracts information and experiences that are familiar. It pulls in thoughts that are congruent with what we already believe. This keeps the mind comfortable. You know how great it feels to have a conversation with someone who believes the same things you do. It validates you and your way of thinking. Will it help you grow? Will it help you make changes? No, not at all. Remember how you used to sit around with certain friends and moan about your weight or the current diet you were on? Did you grow or change? No. If you want to go somewhere other than where you are right now, you will need to prepare yourself to be a bit uncomfortable. You are going to have to change your exposure to conscious information *and* your subconscious "magnet." That self-help book that you read last month and thought was really good is not going to make a bit of difference in your life unless you dig into it and use it in such a way that it shakes up your conscious and subconscious mind.

We recommend that you write in your self-help books and individualize them. Use self-sticking notes to designate powerful passages you want to read again. Cross out every *you* and *we* and insert *I*, then really try the words on for size. Write down important concepts, then write them down again every morning and put them on tape. Look up the words in the dictionary and understand exactly what is being said. You can even create belief statements out of what you are reading and do a whole-brain posture balance for them. Growing, changing, and learning require your participation. Reading about how you'd like to change is better than nothing, but reading alone cannot change things.

Imagining Is Important

It is absolutely impossible to be something you can't imagine. If you cannot even imagine being slim; if you cannot even picture yourself eating small amounts of nutritious foods; if you do not believe that you are a naturally slim person by birth and have all the instincts you need to become slim, then you can't achieve these changes. It is that simple! All the enthusiastic external actions will never stick if the thoughts, beliefs, and images are not there to support them. That is why the mental imaging and the Psych-K we give you are so important. You can learn about food and nutrition and exercise anywhere; we merely included brief information on those subjects for your convenience. It is the conscious and subconscious mind work in this book that will get you where you "ardently desire" to go.

We have become a very literate society. Reading and writing are very highly valued, and we believe that every man, woman, and child should be able to read and write. What we are trying to do when we read and write is to share experiences, thoughts, feelings, and ideas with other people. What we sometimes forget is that words are only as powerful as the meaning they have to the person reading them, and words can often be totally inadequate in what they convey. Try looking at an intricately patterned Oriental rug and describing it in words. The task can be overwhelming. Most of us would say, "Why don't you just send me a picture of it?" This is the reason more and more visual arts are utilized in our society today. Movies, television, and virtual reality are all attempts to convey vivid images from one person to another.

Imaging for Growth and Change. When you want to change the way you think and act, you must be able to imagine it, not just once but at any time, on command. The image must be so available in your mind that when you say the words of your new beliefs, such as "I am naturally slim," the image of what that belief means to you flashes in your mind. The image must be vivid and have a genuine feeling attached to it. It must be accompanied by a feeling of rightness, pleasure, and strength. When someone asks you, "Where would you like to go for lunch?" the images and feelings that flash through your mind in a nanosecond will have to do with the feeling in your stomach, what you had for breakfast, what you have a taste for now, what would be good for your health, and whether following through on these images feels pleasurable or not. You want to think and imagine the same way a slim person does when asked that question.

Psych-K will facilitate changing your subconscious beliefs, which creates the potential to think and act in new ways. However, you will need to give your conscious mind images, patterns, and practice to put this potential into action. Believing that you are a champion tennis player creates the potential to be one. However, if you never pick up a racquet and practice, that potential will remain dormant. The practicing must begin in your mind, before you even step onto the court. Visual imaging, cybernetics, and mental practice are commonplace among top athletes. You can use the same techniques to develop the behavior patterns that enhance your health and slimness.

Framing. The vast majority of people and organizations in our society function on a daily basis out of left-brain logic, order, and language. This includes our educational system. Because of this we have had decades of reinforcement of our verbal abilities and very little support for our imaging abilities. Everyone knows how to image; we do it all day long. However, what you need to know to produce change in your life is how to imagine *purposefully*; how to purposefully develop images in the areas of your life you would like to change, from the way you eat to the job you have. You can devise purposeful images for yourself by taking the words you say and the words you believe and defining them for yourself, making the definitions so detailed that they create a vivid image in your mind. We call this *framing*. It can be fun and is an adventure into yourself and what you really want.

Most people verbalize their wants in very vague terms like "I want to lose some weight," "I want to feel better," or "I want to eat healthier." What do they really mean? What do you mean when you say those things? Do you want to lose weight or release excess fat? How much do you want to release? What is reasonable for your genetic makeup and your weight history? How will you look? Can you imagine your 55-year-old face on a slim body, or are you holding a picture of a 27-year-old in your mind? Can you imagine walking into a grocery store and walking down the produce aisle twice a week? Can you imagine yourself cooking? Sitting down at a table and eating slowly, savoring every bite? These are just a few of the images you need to create to make these things happen for you.

The key is to create the images yourself. My image of savoring a meal will not be yours, though the two may have some things in common. Take one or two key beliefs, like "I am a naturally slim person and I have all of the instincts I need to return to my naturally slim size." Sit down with a dictionary, a pencil, and a sheet of paper. Look up each word in a dictionary or thesaurus, and find the meanings that feel good to you. Then look up the meanings of the words in those definitions. Do this with every word, including the word *I,* which is very powerful and begins every belief statement. You will end up with a strong understanding, consciously and subconsciously, of what you really want.

Next bring in sensory input and write it down:

> *Sight:* What will I and the world around me look like when I act in the manner of my new beliefs?
>
> *Sound:* What will I be saying to myself, and what will others be saying to me?
>
> *Smell:* What smells will I smell when I act in this new way?
>
> *Taste:* What tastes will I taste?
>
> *Touch:* What will I feel on the outside?

Emotions: What will I feel on the inside?

It is rather like creating a collage or putting a puzzle together. You will know when the image is done and when it is firmly a part of you. You will begin to get a *feeling* of pleasure every time you think about your new belief.

Ardently Desiring

Many times we want things, like "losing weight," on a conscious level but are really not sure about it subconsciously. You can ask yourself if you have an ardent, heartfelt desire to become slim and listen for that little voice inside your heart to answer. Or you can muscle-test statements like "I have an ardent desire to become slim and healthy" and "I have very little desire to become slim and healthy." If you test weak to the first or strong to the second, your desires are not supporting your other work and you may indeed end up sabotaging your own efforts at change.

An ardent desire comes from the heart, the spirit, the true self. It is a desire that is grounded in love. Desires grounded in envy, self-loathing, competition, or blame are not desires of the spirit, because they are unloving. Your desire for health and slimness may indeed come from the heart. But it is difficult to have an ardent desire if your mind is filled with fear. When you change, the world around you and all of your relationships change. That can be pretty frightening! When you create the images of yourself as you will be with your new eating habits, imagine how those changes will affect your job, your children, your partner, your parents.

Imagine all the different ways it might affect them, pleasantly or unpleasantly, and then be OK with all of them. Hope for the pleasant ones but know that you will be OK if there are unpleasant ones. If you can be OK with any and all of the reactions you may get, even to the point of knowing what you will say or do, there is absolutely nothing to fear. You can also do a whole-brain posture balance for releasing all the fears connected with people's reactions to your becoming slim.

All of this may seem like a lot of work to you. But remember that work and play can be the same. The feeling you get from doing personal growth work is positive and rewarding, and it is definitely more fun than counting calories.

Nourishment for the Body

Nourishing the spirit and nourishing the mind contribute greatly to the nourishment of the body. Your current body is a physical manifestation of all the thoughts, beliefs, and actions you have taken since the day you were born in perfect physical shape. Each time you take yourself spiritually and mentally closer to your loving, positive nature, your body begins to return to its naturally healthy state. In the beginning of your growth process you may ignore your body while you nourish your spirit and mind. This is OK. Gradually begin to take responsibility for your physical needs as well. Take responsibility for the knowledge and awareness of what is healthy for your body and what is not. The way you eat and exercise are major contributors to your physical health, but they are not the sole contributors. Some people eat fairly well and exercise fairly regularly but participate in health-diminishing activities such as smoking, drinking, drug use, or unprotected sex. It is beyond the scope of this book to address each of these issues specifically. However, the process of growing and changing these habits is almost identical to the one presented here. The habits of getting life priorities straight, developing a sense of purpose and self-love, freeing oneself from judgment, changing the subconscious belief system and nourishing the spirit, mind, and body are part of the process of changing any habit.

Air

Air is a much-ignored but most essential part of nourishing your body. You can survive only a very few moments without it, and yet we all take each breath for granted, sometimes sucking in the most horrendous chemicals or breathing with only the tiniest portion of our upper lungs and chest. Your physical body surrounds your breath, and what and how you breathe are important. Almost every bioenergetic reaction in your body requires the use of oxygen. Breathing deeply and evenly is life-giving and can also be very calming. Look around at the dust and fumes in your environment. Are your lungs constantly having to defend you against an invasion of microorganisms? This can overburden your immune system. Your lungs have an extremely rich supply of blood and absorb both medicine and toxins that are inhaled as rapidly as shooting them into a vein. Investing in filters for your furnace or air filters for your bedroom can be an inexpensive way to improve your health.

Pay attention to how you breathe, at rest and during times of stress. Taking long, slow, deep breaths through your nose, relaxing your abdomen, and using your diaphragm fully relaxes your body and stimulates your circulation. Learn how to breathe this way even during exertion. (*Read Body, Mind and Sport* by John Douillard.)

Water

Water is the next most essential nutrient for the body. Your body is at least 70 percent water, and just staying alive will cause you to lose several quarts a day through your lungs, skin, kidneys, and bowels. This loss must be replaced. The amount of water you need depends on your body size, diet, activity level, and climate. A sedentary person living in a cool climate will require less water than an athlete running in 80-degree heat. Also, a person who eats a lot of fresh fruits and vegetables will glean a lot of water needs from diet and need less actual drinking water. The average daily requirement for water is about three quarts, including food and beverages. However, caffeinated beverages such as coffee, tea, cola, and cocoa, as well as alcoholic beverages, cannot be fully counted as intake because they act as diuretics, increasing water loss through the kidneys. If you have a low caffeine intake and eat some fresh fruits and vegetables, one and a half to two quarts of water should be sufficient.

A lot of people have a poor attitude about drinking plain water, whether it is left over from gulping the recommended amounts on your last diet or just the habit of having to have flavor in beverages. You may want to change your beliefs about water. When you are not well hydrated, all of the following can happen and more: you may increase your food intake, thinking you are hungry when you are really thirsty; the fluid in your joints decreases, causing decreased mobility; you may crave salt and salty foods to help you hold on to the water you have; toxins are not removed efficiently from your body, causing you to feel sluggish and achy; your mucous membranes and skin become dry and are compromised as your first line of defense against infections.

Keep clean filtered water at your desk or wherever you spend a lot of time. Spread your water intake evenly throughout the day. You may want to start the day with a glass or two because you haven't had any water intake during sleep. You also may want to drink a glass an hour before meals, not to fill your stomach but to decrease the odds that you will eat out of thirst instead of hunger. That takes care of one to one and a fourth quarts right there. The rest you can sip on throughout the day. If you sip rather than gulp large amounts, you should have only a minimal increase in your need to use the bathroom. That also normalizes after a few days. Drinking water during meals is not advised because it dilutes the enzymes in your stomach that are necessary for good digestion and it interferes with your ability to assess whether you are satisfied with the amount of food you have eaten. Carbonated beverages also interfere with your ability to assess the hunger signals in your stomach. Frequently drinking fruit juices or sweetened beverages increases your carbohydrate intake tremendously and may elevate your blood sugar and insulin levels in a way that promotes fat storage.

Food

We need food to live. This has always been the dieter's dilemma: "If I just didn't have to deal with food, if I could just stop eating like people stop smoking, I'd be fine." Food is not the enemy;

it is as essential a part of you as air and water. You replace entire organs, bones, blood components, and skin in a matter of months. You are constantly building, breaking down, and building again; thinking, digesting, cleansing all the time. All of this is occurring whether or not you are overweight and whether or not you are exercising. You need a balanced diet of carbohydrates, protein, and fat and a complement of vitamins and minerals even when you are trying to lose excess body fat. An unbalanced diet can lead to the breakdown of proteins and body tissues for energy, leaving you weighing less due to muscle loss along with the fat loss. When you burn your own muscles for fuel, you are destroying the structures that burn fuel and can keep you slim. You want to build muscle, not break it down.

Your body is an energy-consuming machine. Every bodily action from a thought in your head to a bead of sweat on your palm requires energy. You need this energy even when you are overweight. Your body is very efficient. It can break down all three food categories for energy, but it has preferences for energy fuels that make it run more smoothly and efficiently. The order of preference is: (1) carbohydrates, (2) fat available in diet, (3) stored fat, and (4) protein. As you learn to eat only when you're hungry and to balance your intake of carbohydrates, proteins, and fats, your body will begin to dip into its stored fat for energy.

Carbohydrates are a class of food made by green plants in the presence of sunlight. They are literally our way to consume the sun's energy for our own life and growth. Carbohydrates can be classified as *simple* or *complex*. Simple carbohydrates are sugars that break down easily and enter the bloodstream very rapidly. Complex carbohydrates are chains of sugars linked together called *starches*. Complex carbohydrates provide a slower, more even absorption of fuel into the bloodstream. Complex carbohydrates generally contain a nonnutritional substance called *fiber*, which also slows absorption and which is essential for good elimination through the bowels. When complex carbohydrates are refined, such as white flours and pastas and rice, they lose their fiber as well as their vitamins, minerals, proteins, and oils. They become very similar to simple carbohydrates in the way they are absorbed. The rapid absorption of simple and refined carbohydrates can lead to huge shifts in insulin secretion. This excess insulin secretion can cause a precipitous drop in blood sugar, leaving you feeling tired, sleepy, faint, and/or hungry. Insulin also facilitates the storage of fat.

Simple and Refined Carbohydrates	**Complex Carbohydrates**
Cane sugar	Grains and Starch—Wheat,
Fructose	Rye, Buckwheat (whole is best)
Corn syrup	Vegetables—Quinoa, Kasha,
Beet sugar	Oats, Corn, Potatoes
Maple syrup	Rice (brown and wild are best),
Molasses	Barley
Malt sugar (beer and crackers)	Pasta, Bread, Crackers, Chips*
Fruit Juices	Fibrous Vegetables—Asparagus,
	Broccoli, Spinach, Carrots
	Peppers, Cucumbers, Cauliflower
	Onions, Squash, Greens,
	Zucchini, etc.
	Legumes—Beans, Lentils,
	Peas, Peanuts, Soybeans
	Whole Fruits—Apples,
	Berries, Oranges, etc.

*Although pasta, bread, and chips are considered complex carbohydrates, when they're made from white flour they're absorbed by the body the same way sugar is.

For maximum health and slimness, consume as few simple and refined carbohydrates as possible. A balanced intake of complex carbohydrates contains whole grains, legumes, fruits, and vegetables, with an emphasis on fibrous vegetables because of their high-nutrient, high-fiber, low-fat nature.

Fats are the most concentrated form of energy available to us. They contain nine calories for every gram of weight, whereas carbohydrates and proteins contain four calories per gram. A little fat goes a long way! There are several essential fatty acids, sometimes referred to as *vitamin F,* that are absolutely necessary for health. These fats are a component of every cell membrane in the body. You also need a certain amount of fat in your body to protect your internal organs and to keep you warm. The rest of the fat you consume is literally "gravy." You have absolutely no nutritional need for animal fats, which are saturated and contribute to heart disease and cancer. All of the essential fatty acids you need can be obtained from fish and unsaturated plant oils. As you can see in Figure 6, you need just a little bit of fat to grease the wheel of balanced nutrition, and it is best if most of it comes from plant sources.

Just as many simple sugars can be hidden in processed foods, the hidden fat in processed foods, meats, and dairy products can add up to a very large percentage of your intake. Read labels! Nuts and seeds, which are a source of protein, are also a high source of fats even when they haven't been processed in oil. Raw or sprouted nuts and seeds are generally OK if you pay attention to how many you are eating.

Saturated Fats
Meat renderings for gravy
Lard
Butter
Non-Skim Dairy Products:
    Cheese, Cream, Sour Cream
Whole Milk
Coconut Oil, Palm Oil

Unsaturated Fats
Mono—Olive Oil, Canola Oil
Poly—Soybean, Corn, Peanut,
    Sesame, Safflower,
    Cottonseed, etc.

For maximum health and slimness, consume as little saturated fat as possible. Move your fat intake toward monounsaturated oils and those obtained from fish, a teaspoon or two per meal. The Naturally Slim process is aimed at helping you keep enough fat in your diet that you are healthy and don't feel deprived but little enough to encourage your body to use stored body fat for fuel.

Proteins are complex molecules comprising various arrangements of amino acids. They provide the structural matrix for all of your cells, tissues, and organs as well as important messenger molecules such as hormones and neuropeptides. Without protein you wouldn't have a body or a brain. Protein can also be converted to fuel, but it is an energy-consuming process and the body avoids it if at all possible. In the past there was much concern about excessive protein intake by Americans because of the large amounts of meat consumed. However, people have started changing their diets in the interest of health. Those people who have jumped on the high-carbohydrate, low-fat bandwagon or become vegetarians may not be getting enough protein in their diets. An adequate intake of protein is essential for health and imperative for becoming slim. We cannot manufacture protein out of carbohydrates or fats.

Protein does all of the following:

1. It provides the building blocks for antibodies and white blood cells, the core of our immune system.

2. It provides osmotic pressure within blood vessels and cells to keep water from leaking out and causing fluid retention and edema.

3. It provides the building blocks for growth, repair, and maintenance of all cells, tissues, and organs.

4. It increases lean muscle mass in response to exercise, in particular strength training.

5. It can increase your metabolic rate up to 30 percent for several hours after a meal.

Your protein needs vary based on your lean body mass and your activity level and whether you are in a crisis that requires healing or fighting infection. The more active you are or the more involved in exercise, the more building and repair your body needs to do. A range of 0.8 to 1.2 grams of protein per kilogram of slim body weight gives you a ballpark figure (1 kilogram equals 2.2 pounds). In *The Zone*, Barry Sears, Ph.D., provides a very specific way to calculate your protein needs. He tends to favor an even higher protein and lower carbohydrate intake than we do.

Incomplete Proteins
(Must be combined to
    get all eight essential
    amino acids)

Whole Grains
Legumes (Beans, Lentils,
    Peas)
Nuts (⇧fat)
Seeds (⇧fat)

Complete Proteins
(Provide all eight essential
    amino acids)

Fish
Chicken
Turkey
Eggs
Milk /Milk Products (⇧fat)
Meat (⇧fat)
Isolated Protein Powders
    (read label to make sure
    it is complete)

For maximum health and slimness, choose the leanest versions of these proteins as often as possible. Fish, chicken, and turkey are leaner than beef and pork; egg whites are leaner than whole eggs (try mixing two whites and one yolk); dairy products that are skim or 1 percent are leaner than whole-milk dairy products. Whole grains and legumes are leaner than nuts and seeds.

If you are a vegetarian or find it hard to get in a serving of complete protein at every meal, you may want to supplement your protein intake with a protein powder shake of some kind. Get the protein powder at a health food or vitamin store and make your own shake rather than buying the high-carbohydrate, prepackaged instant meal shakes. This way you can make a shake that is balanced and does not have refined sugars or additives.

It is important to increase your lean protein intake when you begin exercising. It is particularly important in strength training because of the muscle tissue that you tear down and rebuild.

Vitamins and minerals are a class of nutrients that are not sources of energy but are essential to both structure and energy production in the body. With the exception of a few of the B vitamins, the body cannot manufacture vitamins or minerals; they must be obtained from diet or supplements. If you are reasonably healthy, eat a balanced sensible diet, and have a lifestyle that is low in stress, you most likely do not need vitamin supplements. How many of you fit into that category? Probably not many. It is beyond the scope of this book to address vitamins and minerals in detail. However, here are three very general recommendations:

1. If you are under the stress of making lifestyle changes and your diet is not the best, consider taking a multivitamin supplement and a separate multimineral supplement. Go to a health food or vitamin store and just ask for a recommendation for a good multivitamin and a good multimineral.

2. If you have not yet incorporated very many whole fruits and vegetables into your meals, take a concentrated fruit and vegetable supplement. These capsules and tablets contain all of the vitamins, minerals, and phytochemicals of five to six servings of fruits and vegetables. Some clients have reported that these supplements eliminate some of their food cravings. This is most likely because the supplement is supplying vital nutrients that are missing from their diet. When you use the fruit and vegetable supplements you get the benefit of the whole dried food in its natural state instead of isolated vitamins and minerals by themselves.

3. If you have sugar cravings or suffer from episodes of low blood sugar, you may benefit from taking the supplement chromium polynicotinate, a mineral found in many fresh fruits and vegetables but often lacking in the typical American diet. Chromium assists in regulating blood sugar levels. It has also been said to

assist in the conversion of fat to muscle. This may be true, but taking chromium will not cancel out food you are eating that contributes to your increased body fat.

If you are interested in knowing more about the health and healing properties of various vitamins and minerals, by all means read up on them. However, if you find yourself spending $100 a month on supplements, you are out of balance! The most important factor in increasing your health and decreasing your excess body fat is to look at your food intake and assess it for quality (Chapter 12) and balance (Chapter 18).

Balance, Balance, Balance

Through the years various and sundry weight loss diets have made various and sundry recommendations for food intake. Some recommend you count only fat grams; some recommend you count carbohydrate grams; some recommend you count calories from all foods. Lately the literature has moved from counting to percentages. *The Zone* recommends a caloric intake that is 30 percent protein, 30 percent fat, and 40 percent carbohydrate for balanced nutrition. Dr. Dean Ornish, author of *Eat More, Weigh Less*, recommends approximately 20 percent protein, 10 percent fat, and 70 percent carbohydrate for balanced nutrition. It can get very confusing.

The fact is, both are correct. One may be right for you, and the other might be right for me. The people who write diet and weight loss books are not out to confuse you or to make you fail. Each book has been written by someone who has experienced genuine success with a certain plan. However, one diet does not fit all. It is more important to focus on what you are doing now and how to make it more healthy than to set goals for grams, percentages, and pounds. Once you start moving toward health and experiencing the positive nature of the changes you have chosen to make, you may want to look at specific percentages and play with them.

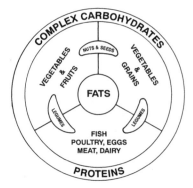

Figure 6. Balanced Nutrition

After you have gotten well into your mind and spirit work, there will come a time when you are ready to begin making changes in the food you eat. You will know it is time when you no longer see good nutrition as something restrictive, like your old diets, but see it as a great way to care for yourself. If you look at the information in this chapter and in Chapter 12 and feel a lot of anger or resistance, it may not be time to change what you are eating. However, it is time to look into that resistance and start doing some belief changes in order to dissolve it and move forward.

When you are ready to start balancing your food intake, we recommend that you follow this six-step process:

1. Know how to recognize carbohydrates, fats, and proteins in your meals.

2. Evaluate your meals and snacks for quality (see Nutrient Density Evaluation Chart in Chapter 12).

3. Evaluate your meals and snacks for balance (see Figure 6 in this chapter).

4. Choose an area of food intake that you are ready to change.

5. Mentally implement the change.

6. Physically implement the change.

We highly recommend increasing the quality of your food intake before you decrease any amounts. If you decrease amounts, and your food quality is poor, you will just become hungrier and more undernourished.

Use the balanced nutrition wheel in Figure 6 as a guideline for a meal or a whole day's worth of meals. You can even look at it as a plate containing a meal made up of two vegetables, a grain, and a protein. Fruits are easily digested and best utilized by the body when eaten in between meals. When fruit is eaten along with or right after a meal, it remains in the stomach juices too long and begins to ferment and form gas in the intestines. Fruit makes a great between-meal snack that can be balanced with a bit of nut butter or a handful of sunflower seeds. That way even your snack is balanced. When you keep your food intake balanced, you keep your body's chemistry in a balance that promotes fat burning rather than fat storage.

Exercise

We are meant to move. Whether you call it *work, play, dance,* or *exercise,* it is all to your benefit. Don't jump into a vigorous program of exercise to "lose weight." Find a combination of strength and endurance activities that you can enjoy for the rest of your life. Exercise is important, but don't start changing so many things in your life at once that you aren't enjoying anything. Use Chapter 13 for information on exercise. Most important, if you have any resistance to exercise, change your beliefs and mental attitude before you make any attempt to incorporate exercise into your life. Willpower cannot take you the distance.

Rest and Sleep

Rest and sleep offer the greatest restorative powers known to us. We need to appreciate that sleep is as much a part of the ebb and flow of a healthy life as exercise. Sleep is our maintenance time. It's when the office is closed and the cleaners, carpenters, and plumbers arrive. They clean up the mental and physical debris of the day and repair and rebuild cells and tissues that are damaged. Just as we would die without air, food, or water, we would die without sleep. Yet many of us act as if sleep is an annoying interference in our lives: "If I just didn't have to sleep, I'd have enough time to do everything." Consider the reverse: If you just didn't do everything, you'd have enough time to sleep! Some overweight people actually feel they don't deserve to rest. They think they should be strapped to some giant treadmill until they burn off all their evil fat. Do you know what naturally slim people do when they are tired? They go to bed. This simple fact can be a startling revelation to those of you who eat at night to stay awake and get things done.

Going to sleep by 10:00 P.M. and arising before 6:00 A.M. corresponds with the natural cycles of your body, according to Ayurveda. Eating lightly in the evening rather than having large, late, heavy dinners will allow you to sleep better. It will also allow your body to concentrate on healing and cleansing instead of digesting food. The middle of the day, between 10:00 A.M. and 2:00 P.M., is the time when your digestion is strongest.

Although America does not recognize siesta time, try to fit in a 15-minute power nap or meditation in the afternoon. It will renew your energy and increase your ability to concentrate. Sometimes a high-protein snack is helpful when you are mentally dragging. Either of these is healthier than hitting the caffeine.

Elimination

Almost as important as the air, food, and water that you put into your body is the flow of waste products and accumulated toxins out of your body. When you breathe polluted air, drink chlorinated water, eat foods that have artificial preservatives and colors, and so on, where do all the toxins go? Hopefully, right back out of your body, but not always, especially if you are not in good physical shape. Your skin, liver, kidneys, and bowels are all organs of elimination. The liver especially works to detoxify substances and then sends them to the bowel for elimination. If you don't have regular elimination patterns, the toxins will remain in your body and be stored, sometimes leading to ill health. In addition, if you don't have a regular pattern of elimination, foods remain in the digestive track too long and start to putrefy and release toxins of their own. If you are drinking sufficient water and eating a healthy volume of whole foods, especially fruits and vegetables, you will generally have little problem with regular elimination, healthy elimination being at least one easily passed stool per day. If this is not happening for you, you may want to consult a health professional for recommendations to increase your regularity and your health.

Some people like to do a specific internal cleansing routine once a season using a special diet or combination of herbs that allows their digestive system to rest and maximum cleansing to occur. If you are interested in this, consult a natural living expert, usually available at your health food store.

Body Therapies—Reaching the Mind and Spirit Through the Body

There are many new and ancient body therapies available today that are nourishing to the body and affect the mind and spirit as well. Having a massage relaxes your body and allows you time to clear your mind and open yourself up to your spirit. Body work can be both physically and mentally healing. We often store the toxic chemicals produced by stress, hate, and anger in the muscles or organs of the body. Gentle manipulation of those areas allows us to release the toxins that can hinder our good health. The following list is just a sample of different types of body work: massage, chiropractic adjustment, reflexology, watsu (a massage and stretch in 94-degree water), Reiki, acupuncture, Rolfing, aromatherapy, Feldenkrais, yoga, tai chi—the list is endless. Explore!

Additional Reading

Nourishment for the Spirit

Adams, Kathleen, M.A. *Journal to the Self.* New York: Warner, 1990.

Chopra, Deepak, M.D. *The Seven Spiritual Laws of Success.* San Rafael: Amber-Allen Publishing and New World Library, 1993.

Dyer, Wayne, Ph.D. *Real Magic.* New York: Harper, 1992.

Kabat-Zinn, Jon. *Wherever You Go, There You Are.* New York: Hyperion, 1994.

Mellin, Laurel, M.A., R.D. *The Solution: 6 Winning Ways to Permanent Weight Loss.* New York: Regan Books, 1997.

Morgan, Marlo. *Mutant Message Down Under.* New York: HarperCollins, 1991.

Thoreau, Henry David. *Walden; or, Life in the Woods.* New York: Dover, 1995.

Nourishment for the Mind

Chopra, Deepak, M.D. *Quantum Healing.* New York: Bantam Books, 1989.

Mellin, Laurel, M.A., R.D. *The Solution—6 Winning Ways to Permanent Weight Loss.* New York: Regan Books, 1997.

Moyers, Bill. *Healing and the Mind.* New York: Doubleday, 1993.

Naparastek, Belleruth. *Staying Well with Guided Imagery.* New York: Warner Books, 1994.

Oslander, Sheila, and Lynn Schrader. *Superlearning 2000.* New York: Delacorte Press, 1994.

Roger, John, and Peter McWilliams. *You Can't Afford the Luxury of a Negative Thought.* Los Angeles: Prelude Press, 1988.

Nourishment for the Body

Braly, James, M.D. *Dr. Braly's Food Allergy and Nutrition Revolution*. New Canaan: Keats, 1992.

Chopra, Deepak, M.D. *Perfect Weight*. New York: Harmony Books, 1994.

Diamond, Harvey, and Marilyn Diamond. *Fit for Life II*. New York: Warner Books, 1987.

Haas, Elson M., M.D. *Staying Healthy with Nutrition*. Berkeley: Celestial Arts, 1992.

Kamen, Betty, Ph.D. *The Chromium Connection*. Novato: Nutrition Encounter, 1990.

Landis, Robyn. *Body Fueling*. New York: Warner Books, 1994.

Sears, Barry, Ph.D. *The Zone*. New York: Regan Books, 1995.

Somer, Elizabeth, M.A., R.D. *Nutrition for Women*. New York: Henry Holt, 1993.

Townsley, Cheryl. *Food Smart*. Colorado Springs: Pinon Press, 1994.

A Special Note About Weight Loss

Last night I had a dream. I was riding the sub-way, and I had lost 56 pounds. I checked the Lost and Found Department, and much to my dismay it was there and I was forced to claim it.

JUST IN CASE there is any doubt in your mind, whenever we use the term *weight loss* in this book we are not talking about losing and we are not really talking about weight. Weight loss could be water, fat, muscle, or an amputated arm or leg. They all weigh something, and they all register the same when you get on the scale. However, a pound of muscle lost is a tragedy, and so is the loss of an arm or a leg. Water loss may be healthy if you are retaining excess water. What you are really concerned with is excess body fat, and you want to release it, not lose it. Losing things triggers an automatic response to find them again; you don't feel right until you do. Or you become sad and go into mourning for whatever is lost for good. What you really want is the healthy release of excess body fat for energy. Fat is not bad; it is merely energy in stored form. You don't need to lose it; just transform it into usable energy.

Natural Release of Excess Fat

On your journey to natural slimness you will experience a very different pattern of fat release from any you have ever had before. It is subtle and gentle, it preserves muscle, and it is permanent! Forget the way you looked when you were losing weight on your last diet. At that time your body was in starvation mode and selected certain pockets of fat over others because they were the least important. When becoming naturally slim you may first lose fat that is not even visible—the excess around your body organs. You may see your neck and face become slimmer before your tummy. Your fingers may become slim before your shoulders. The pattern is different for everyone, but the amazement is the same. One day you find your spring clothes are looser than last season. Or you are getting dressed to go out and put on a necklace that used to be tight and realize it isn't tight anymore.

As stated earlier in the book, we recommend that you don't weigh yourself. If you must measure something, find someone who can measure your body fat percentage for you. The best thing to do is just to feel the fit of your clothes. Have you ever experienced a feeling of lightness, energy, and vitality and gotten on the scale, only to find the number unchanged and your vitality gone in an instant? Don't let a number on a metal box dictate the amount of enjoyment you get out of life. Don't give away your sense of purpose and fulfillment to a scale or a tape measure. The key to enjoying the process of becoming naturally slim is to get deeply involved in the process of life and health and not to focus on the outcome, the pound, the percentage, or the dress size. Have a picture of yourself in your mind that is naturally slim, but release the need to measure and compare. If you are living this journey to slimness every day, you are going to feel wonderful, and you will not need a scale to tell you so.

Even after all I have said to you about focusing on the process and not the pounds, there is still most likely a nagging thought in the back of your mind about how much weight you will lose and how fast. In order to quiet that thought I will give you some data about what we have seen so far. Clients who stay consistently in the process have experienced an approximate weight loss of 6 to 12 pounds per year. This an average, not a guarantee. In some of our clients the weight loss is a steady one or two pounds per month. In others the weight loss has occurred in clumps, such as five pounds in one week and then none for six months, or 10 pounds in one month and none for the rest of the year.

Addressing weight loss in terms of years may come as a shock. It is important to remember that with the 10 habits of naturally slim people you are choosing gradual, permanent weight loss instead of a temporary quick fix. We caution you not to judge yourself against any standard but yourself. The steadier your commitment is to daily personal growth work, the steadier your fat release will be. However, everyone's journey will be different. Your fat release will also depend on your history. It will be slower if you've been a chronic dieter. It will also be slower if you have a lot of emotional issues wrapped up with your fat. There are also genetic factors and your body type and metabolism to consider. Rather than try to figure out where you should be, do what you need to do to move toward health and slimness. If you are enjoying every day of your life, what else could you desire?

Body Type and Metabolism

Although we like to consider each person an individual, it is sometimes helpful to point out similarities among us. We have found this extremely valuable in helping people understand the characteristics of their body type and what type of body they can realistically image as their naturally slim body. Everyone who is naturally slim is not the same size! We have a distorted view of what our bodies should look like because of the predominance of one particular body type portrayed in the media. We look to magazines and TV to define normal and natural instead of observing the normal, natural people around us.

There are three basic body types that have been referred to in Ayurveda for thousands of years and in America for the better part of a century. Ayurveda names them Kapha, Pitta, and Vata. Western science names them endomorph, mesomorph, and ectomorph. Few people will fit neatly into one body type, and Ayurveda actually names 10 variations on the basic three body types. What we want to do is give you a general feel for body types. We want you to know that there is more than one type of normal body. When everyone is at his or her naturally slim best, there will still be people who are larger than fashion models. It's their nature, and most likely it is your nature also. People who are of a larger, metabolically slower body type are the people who also gain weight easily. People who are slender, with high metabolic rates, are less likely to gain weight. It's not unfair; it just is. It is no reason to abandon your journey to health.

In the following chart we have listed some of the general physical, hunger, and exercise characteristics for these three basic body types. When you look at the characteristics to see where you fit, keep in mind that these characteristics describe your body *before* you accumulated your excess body fat, *before* you had been on numerous diets. You may find that you fit in one type or another or you may fit in between types. Ayurvedic medicine describes an entire set of personality and mental functions that generally go with each body type, and you may look them up in one of the additional readings if you are interested. Above all, remember that all three are normal, natural body types and that Type I bodies are not supposed to be trying to be Type IIs and Type III bodies are not supposed to be trying to be Type Is.

Every one of our clients has been either Type I or Type II. Type IIIs generally are such fast food burners that they rarely gain weight. They tend to be those people you envy who can eat anything they want and not gain weight. They may not gain weight, but their health and energy suffer tremendously when they eat in an out-of-balance manner.

Two other interesting body typing systems, both based on glandular function and fat distribution, have also been published: *The Body Shaping Diet* by Dr. Sandra Cabot and *Dr. Abravanel's Body Type Diet* by Elliot D. Abravanel, M.D. If you read these

Type I	Type II	Type III
Soft, rounded figure	Muscular, stocky	Lean, frail
Large frame, fleshy	Medium frame	Fine bones/long limbs
Solid, strong build	Medium build, strong	Light thin build
Veins and tendons well covered	Veins fairly prominent	Veins and tendons very prominent
Muscles developed, but covered	Muscles build easily	Building muscles difficult
Slow graceful movements	Strong, efficient stride	Fair endurance
Good endurance	Medium endurance	Energy comes in bursts
Steady energy	Energy very dependent on food intake	Irregular digestion
Slow digestion	Strong digestion	Very fast food burner
Slow food burner	Fast food burner	Irregular hunger
Mild hunger signals	Sharp hunger and thirst	Tends to overexert/tire
Gains weight easily	Perspires easily	Body fat fairly even distribution
Carries extra weight in hips, thighs, and lower abdomen	Carries extra weight between shoulders and hips	Rectangular shape
Percent body fat high normal	Legs remain slim	Percent body fat low normal
Difficulty losing weight, even when follows a diet to the letter	Percent body fat mid-normal	Rarely gains weight
When out of balance, craves creamy and/or spicy foods	Loses weight fairly easy when following a diet	When out of balance, craves sweets or doesn't eat
	When out of balance craves sweets, starches, and caffeine	

books, read them for body typing information and general food guidelines only. Steer clear of the diet mentality. Several people we know have really "found themselves" as one of these body types and were thrilled to realize what foods might specifically be contributing to their problems. Others have found that reading them just added to their general confusion about what to eat. When in doubt, return to your own wisdom. Choose quality and balance, and you can't go wrong.

Be at peace with whatever body type your spirit resides in. Know that you can be healthy and slim whatever type you are. You can improve your digestion, your metabolism, your endurance and strength, and be the best "you" you can be instead of the best someone else. You can do this by coming into balance, which means coming to know your true self, not some media image you thought you had to be.

Additional Reading

Chopra, Deepak, M.D. *Perfect Weight*. New York: Harmony Books, 1994.

Douillard, John. *Body, Mind and Sport*. New York: Crown, 1994.

TWENTY

Embracing the Process of Growth and Change

There really is no such thing as standing still in life. You are either moving forward or sliding back. Growth is the natural state of all living things.

TO THOSE OF YOU who took our suggestion and are reading this chapter first, welcome. To those of you who are reading this chapter last, welcome. Whether this is the first chapter or the last, it is the beginning. Becoming slim is about making changes. Not just changes in what you eat but also changes in the way you live your life in body, mind, and spirit. Not change for the sake of change, but personal growth, moving forward. Not just a change in dress size in time for the class reunion but instead a blueprint to build on for the rest of your life. In the past your weight loss efforts were probably fairly intense and punitive. This time if you choose to use this book as a guide, you will embark on a gentle upward cycle in your life that will buoy your spirit, clear your mind, and lead you to a naturally slim body.

In the first chapter of this book we presented the downward spiral of diet mentality. Continuing on this spiral leads to physical and mental ill health, and in the case of bulimics and anorexics it can actually lead to death. Getting into the upward spiral of growth and change can lead to physical and mental wellness and ultimately life. Yes, life as in the statement "Get a life." Stop dabbling on a canvas of despair and paint yourself a masterpiece. Leading a life of happiness, health, and fulfillment is the journey of a master, a journey that is never really completed because there will always be something more to learn or a new way to do an old thing, places to go, and things to be. If you think your life is going to be magically better when you become slim, you have it backward: make your life magically better, and the slim body will follow. Don't set timetables for yourself. Change and growth follow what I call "universe time"—that is, they happen when the time is right. Human beings invented calendars and clocks in an attempt to understand and measure the immeasurable. That is infinity. Time can mark the coming and going of the natural cycles of the moon and the seasons, but it cannot mark when a spirit is ready to change and grow.

If you were a simpler form of life, say a tomato plant, we could predict more accurately the path of your growth. But even then the weather, the amount of watering and weeding that is done, and all kinds of things could make our predictions inaccurate. Anyway, you are not a tomato plant; you are a very complex, three-dimensional human being. That is why you require more than a blanket prescription for diet and exercise.

Developing an understanding of the growth process is important for your journey. Embracing the growth process and being OK with its ups and downs and ins and outs is essential. If you understand and embrace the process, we will be able to assist you in developing your own personal path toward health and slimness.

Feelings—Your Entry into the Process

Entry into the growth process often occurs when intense feelings tap your inner self on the shoulder, saying, "Please notice me—something is wrong." Feelings are extremely important. Hiding your feelings, ignoring them, blaming other people for them, or stuffing them down with a bowl of chocolate ice cream thwarts

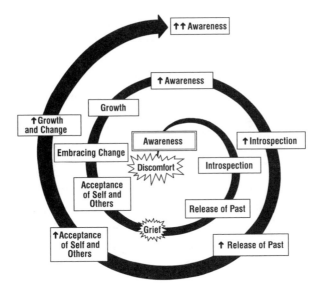

Figure 7. The Upward Spiral of Growth and Change

the wonderful mission those feelings were on when they bubbled up from the depths of your soul. "Wonderful mission?" you ask. "How can feeling rotten, depressed, and unhappy be wonderful?" Here is how. As we've said, you were born happy, joyful, curious, willing, deserving, loving, trusting, and bursting with self-esteem. You ran your physical body based solely on your natural instincts instead of the advice and opinions of others. These are your spiritual qualities. These are your birthright. When you were born, your spiritual qualities were expressed in every belief, thought, and action you undertook. Right now you are in a very different physical form, and you have accumulated millions of beliefs and thoughts, but those spiritual qualities are still in there. Those qualities are an inner flame, a pilot light that never goes out. When you think thoughts or take actions that are in opposition to those positive qualities, you experience discomfort, unhappiness, and conflict. Most people enter the process of growth and change because they acknowledge those feelings and want something different.

Whenever you have uncomfortable feelings, begin to look at them without judgment. People sometimes say to themselves: "I have everything I could ever want. I have no reason to be unhappy, but I am." "I have such a wonderful job. I shouldn't be angry at my boss, but I am!" These are judgments about feelings. Feelings are not good or bad, right or wrong; they just are. And they are very helpful to us if we see them as messengers and not as something awful. To feel is to be alive. To feel discomfort and to listen to it is to grow. Sit with your feelings, allow them to flow through you, and then ask your inner self, "What can I learn from this? What am I thinking or doing that is causing my inner self to cry out for attention?" If you don't get an answer right then, know that you will in time and just stay in the process of growth and change.

Once you have entered the process and are working on a particular life change, you may uncover other areas of your life that call for your attention. For instance, you may enter the growth process totally aware that you are miserable because you are 50 pounds overweight and then find out along the way that the reason you are overweight is to protect yourself from close relationships. At that point your growth work needs to be in the area of feeling safe around people, not a new exercise regime. The tools offered to you in this book concerning belief changes and Psych-K are as valuable to you in changing your beliefs about relationships as they are in changing the types of food you eat.

Being overweight is a symptom of one or more areas of imbalance in your life. It is not strictly a function of diet and exercise. Be careful not to be overwhelmed by all your self-discovery. Work in one area of your life at a time. Even though it may seem that what you're working on has nothing to do with your weight, it does. Any area of your life that becomes more balanced will contribute to your ability to follow your natural instincts. Focus on the process, not the goal. Stay off that bathroom scale!

Awareness or Consciousness

Simply feeling unhappy or uncomfortable does not mean you are on the path of growth and change. Often people choose to sit and wallow in their feelings for hours, days, or years. The key to moving forward is to step out of the feeling, own it, and be willing to do something about finding its cause. Stepping outside your physical and mental feelings and into your true self, inner self, or higher self is called *awareness* or *consciousness*. It is a wake-up call. A wake-up call can be caused by something life threatening, like a car accident, or by something minor, such as a pair of pants that are too tight to get into. Both situations trigger feelings, and you can be aware of those feelings and use them as a springboard to growth and change or just feel bad and pass up the opportunity.

The intensity of the event does not determine what any one individual will do. Hearing the wake-up call and taking positive action is the important part. Many of us have become so numb and unaware of what is happening to us that we stop running on our treadmill only when we land flat on our backs, physically ill. Even then, most people do not take the time to examine what got them into the situation. They just want the doctor to fix it so that they can get back on the treadmill. This is where many people turn to quick fixes. All they know is that they are in pain and they want to feel better as soon as possible. Quick fixes offer temporary relief. Permanent change requires movement to the next stage, introspection.

Awareness is a nonjudgmental state. We see the situation for exactly what it is without guilt or blame. Being awake, being aware, feeling feelings, and hearing an inner voice are key to the process of growth and change. Becoming aware of the thoughts and feelings you have about your body and eating and becoming aware of how you care for yourself in times of stress or anger are important to making lasting changes in your life. Much of the information and many of the exercises in this book focus on awareness. Practicing awareness is fun, and the more you do it on a moment-by-moment, day-by-day basis, the better you will become at it. I don't know about you, but I would much rather hear whispers than wailing sirens for my wake-up calls.

Introspection or Self-Examination

Self-examination, thinking about one's own thoughts and attitudes, is a uniquely human process. We are the only animals here on earth who are capable of looking into ourselves. Introspection is a skill that is used over and over again in the process of growth and change. If the mere thought of getting to know yourself scares you or you find yourself saying, "This is garbage; I can lose weight without all this introspection stuff," we hear you! We've been in that spot exactly! We've dumped the introspection and lost weight on another food plan, *and* we've gained it all back and more. Reconsider, keep reading, and balance for the belief "Looking deeply into my own feelings, thoughts, and beliefs is safe and healthy."

To participate fully in your own growth process, you must accept two truths: (1) You cannot grow or change any person but yourself. (2) What you believe and what you think have a direct influence on what you do and how you feel. During introspection you take a look at who you are, what you think and believe that is causing you to act in ways that make you unhappy. What is the true nature of your body? Your mind? Your spirit? What do you really want? Peel your feelings like an onion. Pull off layer after layer, asking yourself, "Why?" and "What then?" Find out what is at the core of those feelings. What is it you really want?

Often what people who "want to lose weight" really want is attention from other people, love, security, admiration, happiness, and other things that really are not connected to the size of the body. It is their feelings and perceptions about the world that cause them to feel devoid of love and happiness. Many overweight people are looking for validation and acceptance from others to make them happy when what they really need to do is validate and accept themselves.

During this time of self-examination, begin to decide what you want to end and what you want to begin. Weigh the pluses and the minuses of the endings and the beginnings to make the decision to move forward or stay the same. Think about how your change will affect the people around you. Putting your own pluses and minuses on a piece of paper can be very helpful. You may on the surface think, Well, for heaven's sake, there are no minuses to becoming slim. Believe me, if you did not have your very own set of minuses for being slim, you would have done it a long time ago. The following list contains a sample of some of the minuses our clients have come up with. If I get slim . . . .

> I will attract men's/women's attention, and I won't know how to handle it.
>
> I won't have an excuse for not doing all those things I've been waiting to do until I get slim.
>
> People will expect more from me.
>
> I'll be tempted to cheat on my husband/wife/lover.
>
> I'll feel small, naked, vulnerable, unprotected.
>
> What will I do with all the time I spend complaining and obsessing about my body and the food I put into it?
>
> I'll be rejected by my overweight friends.

What are your reasons for staying overweight or not becoming slim? Try sitting in whole-brain posture and ask yourself that question. You'll be surprised by how you answer.

Endings

To clear the path for growth and change, we must choose to end certain beliefs, thoughts, and actions, specifically the ones that are producing our unhappiness. The endings we must make come from the introspection we have done. If we are trying to rush through the process of growth and change without sufficient introspection, we may try to end things that are unrelated to our core issues, the ones that caused the feelings that sent us into the process in the first place. In the arena of becoming naturally slim, it is much more important to end self-hate than to end your consumption of high-fat foods. In fact, ending self-hate may assist you to end all kinds of self-defeating behavior.

People tend to try to skip this step and go directly to new beginnings, new habits, and new foods. They think they can just begin new habits, and those will replace the old ones. Here is where the breakdown occurs in your usual way of making changes. *Your old habits and behaviors were developed for a reason. They met a certain need that you have. If you do not discover the reasons for the habit and meet the need in some other way, you will be unable to end the old habit. You cannot pick up and hold on to a new habit unless you let go of the old and all the reasons you needed it.*

Imagine you are standing in the park and in your cupped hands you hold a giant pinecone that gives you great pleasure. A little way down the path you spot a golden egg. With great admiration, holding tightly on to your pinecone, you rush up to the golden egg. "Wow," you say. "I'd really like to have that egg." You look at it, you covet it, but you really don't think it's yours or that you deserve to find such a beautiful treasure. Or maybe you aren't sure it will really bring you the joy you think it will or you fear that people will want it or try to steal it from you. You look at your pinecone, and it is a sure thing. You've had it for years, and it brings you pleasure. Finally, after trying to find out if anyone in the area lost the golden egg, you decide you really truly want it. *But to pick up the golden egg, you must put down the pinecone.* No matter how little value the pinecone may have in and of itself, it still will be perceived as something given up, something lost, and you will grieve for it when you begin to put it down.

It is the same with habits. Picking up the new habit is not the hard part; it is letting go of the old. With every sense of loss we go through a mini–grieving process until we are able to truly see the event as one of change and growth instead of loss.

Grieving

A universal process of grief was described by Elisabeth Kübler-Ross in her classic book *On Death and Dying*. When I read that book in nursing school, I had no idea of the widespread application it might have in life. I brushed it aside and figured that when someone I know dies, I'll look it up. But grieving has to do with a sense of loss whether real or perceived, and it does not apply only to the loss of a beloved human being. It applies to any perceived loss—of a person, an animal, an arm or a leg, or an unborn child. It could be divorcing the spouse that beat you; it could be leaving home to go to college; it could even be losing the habit of stuffing yourself with food at night to relieve the stresses of the day. Any perceived loss will be grieved in various stages until you can come to a resolution that you, as a person, are whole and OK without the person, limb, or habit that is gone.

The amount of time it takes to go through the grieving process is very different for every person. It can range from seconds in the case of a belief you are balancing for, to years for people who choose to stay stuck. Grieving has several stages, all of which we go through, whether we do it fast or slow. The length of time spent at each stage is not important. What's important is to move through and not get stuck at any stage. If you are aware that you feel a sense of loss and you are knowledgeable about the grieving process, you can give yourself a nudge when you find yourself stuck. Many people involved in life changes get stuck in denial, anger, and blaming. To move out of any stage that you are stuck in, you must be aware that you are stuck.

Stages of Grief

Denial. At this stage you try to protect your inner nature by denying that you even have a problem or that you are feeling bad or that you need to stop doing or thinking something that has been part of your lifestyle for years. There is a new group of people that has emerged out of the ranks of chronic dieters, and they are the people that I refer to as "obese and happy." They proclaim that they love and accept themselves exactly as they are (which is good) and that they intend never to concern themselves with weight again. This is fine for strong, healthy people who may be 20 or 30 percent over their naturally slim weight. But to be 100 or 200 pounds overweight and be perfectly happy to stay there is saying, "I am perfectly happy dying younger. I'm perfectly happy eating foods that create ill health and excess fat. I am perfectly happy with my thighs rubbing together when I walk and being unable to sit in a chair at the movie theater."

If in their heart and soul they can truthfully say those things, then bless them. More likely they are denying their problems because they can no longer stand the pain. They shouldn't feel bad about themselves, but they do not need to limit their potential for health either. They too are naturally slim by birth. However, like all of us, they are frustrated because the only way they know to deal with their weight is the unsuccessful, unhappy adventure of dieting. "Obese and happy" people have taken the most important step in the process of becoming naturally slim, and that is to accept themselves exactly the way they are. The rest of the process is there for them whenever they are ready.

Anger and Blaming. At this stage you are angry that you have come to this place of loss and discomfort, and you look for persons, places, and things to blame. Taking responsibility for yourself at this point is too painful. It is much easier to blame your weight on your mother, your father, the media, or the diets you've been on than to say, "I, _____ [insert name], am fatter than I care to be for my health and other reasons. I am this way because I chose to use ice cream to comfort myself; I chose to continue to diet even when it was making me fatter; I chose to eat second helpings even when I was not at all hungry; I chose to eat the dinner my mother-in-law so kindly made so as not to hurt her feelings. I made those choices because I thought they were the best thing to do at the time. Now I want to make different choices based on new knowledge and beliefs."

Were you a "bad" person then? Are you a better person now? The answer to both is no. There is no blame; there is no guilt; there just is the past and how it was then and the present and how it is now. Many people get stuck at this stage, especially in their anger and blaming of parents, spouses, handicaps, the diet industry, etc. They think self-responsibility will be painful, but it doesn't have to be if guilt is removed and forgiveness takes its place.

Bargaining. At this stage you make a last-ditch effort to avoid the perceived pain of ending and taking self-responsibility. You make bargains with yourself and higher powers or jump into a quick fix to cover the pain or return to the denial that you have any problem at all. Staying at this stage, trying to wiggle out of moving forward, can delay the grieving process as well as the over-all process of growth and change.

Acceptance and Emotional Release. At this stage of grieving you finally break through all barriers and accept the ending as truth. Part of you is gone, whether it is a loved one, a pet, or a habit. Holding on to it has no more positive benefits for you. You truly accept the ending with all of its pluses and minuses, and there is usually a very strong emotional release that accompanies this—crying, elation, remorse. As you move out of your grief, you move back into the main spiral of positive growth and change.

Acceptance of Self and Others. Accepting yourself and others and taking responsibility for your own life involves forgiveness. At this stage you become able to forgive yourself the past and forgive others who may have treated you unlovingly. You can realize that you did the best you could do at the time and so did they. Holding on to anger and blame can only hold you back. When you forgive yourself and others for all the unhealthy things you did in the past, you can move forward. Holding on to guilt, anger, and blame holds you back. Forgiveness and letting go are extremely freeing. It feels like an enormous weight has been lifted from your heart. Though forgiving yourself may bring tears, the feeling afterward can be light and giddy. Enjoy this stage. Feel the feelings; know where you got those feelings. You got them from spending time on your own personal growth. You can feel that way a lot more often. When you are no longer tethered to the past with fear, guilt, and blame, you stand clearly in your true self and the present moment. That is why this stage feels so good.

This stage of recovery can be exhilarating and comfortable. It feels so pleasurable after the feelings of grief and loss that many people get stuck here. Even though we know that 12-step programs have helped millions of people, it bothers us to hear people refer to themselves as recovering alcoholics after 25 years without alcohol in their life or to know people who make recovery groups their life and attend them three, four, or five times a week. We would like to see a 13th step that releases these people to be free from their past and move on.

Know what stage you are at in your personal growth process. Be aware of when you are stuck and when you are ready to move on. Then give yourself some new beliefs and mental images that will support your movement to the next stage. If you just remain recovered from the old but not committed to the new for too long, your growth process will stall.

Embracing Change

When you embrace change, you actually walk forward to meet it with loving, open arms. You take it to your heart and have a genuine desire to seek it out and nurture it. You feel committed to being or doing something differently. This is not willpower. When you are holding on to all of your old habits and fears and angers, you need willpower. When you have come through the process of growth step by step and recognize, forgive, and release all those old feelings and habits, you have a natural desire to move forward.

It is the "fire in the belly" feeling you may get about a certain cause, like your life's work, your children, clean water, or food for the hungry. It is a fire in the belly about your own health and wellness, in spirit, mind, and body. This is a commitment to a new beginning and whatever it takes to succeed. A feeling of no turning back. A commitment to learning new theories and practicing new techniques. A realization that you must take an active part in your own growth. A state of openness and willingness to hear new ideas and try new theories, knowing you are on your way to your goal and if one way doesn't work you'll find another.

Just being aware and not acting on that awareness will not produce growth. Conversely, just acting without the supporting awareness and process will also not produce growth. Many of us have a heck of a time making commitments for many reasons. Being stuck in the process of growth may mean being unable to make a commitment, whether it be a commitment to take the time you need to do the practices in this book or a commitment to find out what healthy food is and at least bring it into the house. The inability to make a commitment, to one small step at a time, is another tap on the shoulder for you. It is a new awareness. Take your newfound awareness into the spiral of growth and find out why you can't make the commitment to something you really want. One of the most common reasons and the root of many issues we have is self-love and self-trust. If you really loved yourself, you would find the time to do loving things for yourself. If you really loved and trusted yourself, you would take the risk of trying this new approach and know that you would be OK whether it worked for you or not.

"Isn't loving yourself vain and selfish? Aren't we supposed to put others first?" Always putting others' needs before your own because you "should" misses the spirit of the act. The goal is to be able to spontaneously and lovingly recognize other people's needs. This can happen only when you genuinely love yourself and meet your own needs for love so regularly that you overflow with love and generosity. Don't put the cart before the horse. Be aware that you may be in a codependent pattern of behavior. Ask yourself, "Do I help everyone else and solve everyone else's problems at the expense of my own well-being? Do I often feel like a martyr, as if the whole world benefits while I become more and more miserable?" If you answer yes, you may benefit from reading a short book called *Codependence* by Anne Wilson Schaef. This pattern of behavior is common among women and caregivers. It ultimately leads to that exhausted, burned-out "I have nothing left to give" feeling you may be experiencing. Recognizing the pattern and letting it go may be one of the biggest steps you can take toward becoming naturally slim.

Growth—From Seed to Blossom and Back

There is a universal cycle of growth and change among all living things. Even though we humans add our own unique qualities of introspection and emotional attachment, we can learn from the cycles in nature. We can look to plants, insects, and animals, and find over and over the cycle of growth and change. The tiny brown seed that we hold in our hand represents unlimited potential, all of our dreams and desires. When we come through the stages of awareness, introspection, letting go, and acceptance, we are preparing ourselves to truly own those seeds, those wants and dreams and desires, and to take responsibility to do something with them. When we embrace the process of change, we place the seed in the ground and give it what it needs to grow. For the seed it is good soil, water, sunshine, and as few weeds as possible. For us it is choosing new beliefs and thoughts, imaging our desires, pulling out the weeds of negative thoughts, and knowing that the seed will grow. Above ground, it may look as if nothing is happening, but underneath a miracle is taking place. This is the most important and tumultuous stage of all. This is the stage where the action is! We are learning, practicing, falling down, getting up, finding more things that need to be changed, reaching forward into new beliefs and beginnings, and falling backward into depression, bargaining, anger, and blame. The seed at this stage is developing the root system it needs to support a full-grown plant.

This is the part of the process that requires understanding and faith. It is important to understand how the growth process works so that you can be in it and know that you are OK, no matter where you are in it. It requires faith in that you continue to feed yourself spiritual, mental, and physical nourishment, even when it doesn't look as if anything is happening. Your spiritual and mental growth may not be immediately visible, but if you stay in the process there is no way that that you can avoid seeing the results. Just as you have faith that each seed you plant will grow and blossom into the plant it is destined to be, have that faith in yourself. Do you dig up a seed to make sure it is growing? Do you open up a cocoon to see if the butterfly is done yet? If you do, the plant or butterfly may die. Banish the doubts in your mind. They will slow you down and keep you from realizing your full potential.

At some point during your growth a body, mind, and spirit connection takes place that incorporates your efforts as true change. You are no longer the same; you think differently. It's kind of like when you are learning a foreign language and you have drilled and practiced and read, and one day you wake up and are thinking in French or German. The belief, thoughts, and action patterns that you have been nurturing start to flow effortlessly. I will never forget the first time I looked in the refrigerator when I was feeling depressed and my very own head said to me, "There is absolutely nothing in there that will help you feel better" and I walked away. I knew at that moment it was all worthwhile. To be able to automatically think the thoughts of a naturally slim person was awesome. All of my watering and weeding had paid off. My seeds were blossoming.

Just as the flower of change blossoms, it also scatters the seeds of new awareness that send us back to the growth process, and life goes on, a continuing upward spiral of growth and consciousness. Your journey toward becoming naturally slim will scatter seeds of awareness in many areas of your life. Take advantage of them, nurture them, and continue to create your life garden.

Additional Reading

Covey, Stephen. *The 7 Habits of Highly Effective People*. New York: Fireside Press, 1990.
Leonard, George. *Mastery*. New York: Plume, 1991.

About the Authors

Jill H. Podjasek, M.S., R.N., founder of the Center for Positive Life Changes, teaches classes and workshops on becoming Naturally Slim.

Jennifer Carney is in private practice as a personal change coach and a motivational speaker. Both live in Denver, Colorado.

If you have any questions about *The Ten Habits of Naturally Slim People* or would like information about upcoming Naturally Slim seminars, classes, or workshops, please send a self-addressed stamped envelope to:

> The Center for Positive Life Changes
> PO Box 100157
> Denver, CO 80250
> or
> E-mail: Natslim@aol.com

Index